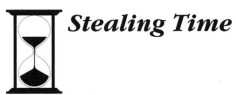

Stealing Time

Stealing Time:

The New Science of Aging

Fred Warshofsky

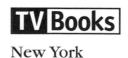

New York

Cataloging-in-Publication Data
Warshofsky, Fred.
    Stealing time : the new science of aging / Fred Warshofsky. — 1st ed.
    p. cm.
    Includes bibliographical references and index.
    ISBN: 1-57500-045-8
    1. Aging. I. Title.
  QP86.W37 1999   612.6'7
                             QBI99-451

All photographs courtesy of Rubin Tarrant Productions/PBS.

TV Books, L.L.C.
1916 Broadway, Ninth Floor
New York, NY 10019
www.tvbooks.com

Interior design by Rachel Reiss
Manufactured in the United States of America

For Brian and Adrian and
Jeffrey and Michael—the first
generation to benefit fully
from the new science of aging.
Lechayim!

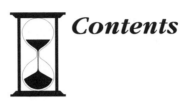# Contents

Introduction: The New Science of Aging   9

1. The Aging Paradox   19

2. Other Species   47

3. The Genetics of Aging   71

4. Extending Life   103

5. Exercise and Hormones   135

6. Mastering the Mind   167

7. Alzheimer's and the Chemistry of the Aging Brain   197

8. Tomorrow   227

   Bibliography   233

   Index   237

Introduction: The New Science of Aging

We are witnessing the birth of a revolutionary new science—the science of aging. It will challenge our beliefs and may grant us the dream of enduring youth. It will also present us with a set of challenges unlike any in human history. In some instances it will offer almost God-like powers, the ability to literally double the Biblical allotment of three score and ten, and the possibility of remaking the genetic map of the individual and eliminating many of the diseases of aging that have afflicted humans since the dawn of time.

How we as a nation respond to these challenges, both ethical and social, will determine the quality of life not only for the elderly, but also for everyone in the new millennium. What uses we make of these newly doubled life spans will challenge our imaginations and the very best qualities we like to think of as human. The consequences of too many elderly, putting demands on too little money and too few facilities, the problems of paying for Social Security and Medicare—these are but the immediate and obvious problems that will be posed by the new and largest generation in history of the oldest old.

Indeed, the most common fear running through all discussions on aging is the presumed staggering economic burden an exploding population of aging baby-boomers would create. But research into the actual costs of caring for and treating the oldest old has revealed some surprising and encouraging trends. A 1995 study by the Health Care Financing Administration calculated that medical expenditures for the last two years of life average $22,600 for people who die at seventy, but a mere $8,300 for those who live to be one hundred.

And the cost of medical care will drop even further as the baby-boom generation grows old. The net result will be to ease pressure on Medicare and the fears that it will go bankrupt under an avalanche of claims from hordes of sick and infirm, aging baby-boomers. A study co-authored by H. Dennis Tolley, professor of statistics at Brigham Young University, and six other researchers suggests that improved medical technology could eventually lower total health-care costs and even boost the economy. "Most people become eligible for Medicare when they turn sixty-five," explains Tolley. "From that point, a person who lives to be ninety will incur less overall health-care costs than a person who lives to be seventy-five, even though the first person lived fifteen years longer," says Tolley.

The new science of aging has revealed many more surprises, forever altering our traditional views of aging. A host of "givens" are proving to be no more than shibboleths swept aside by the new research, replaced by facts and ideas that were not even suspected or dreamed of ten or fifteen years ago. In one sense, the revolution we are witnessing will in its ultimate implications be as important as the scientific watersheds marked by Mendel's articulation of the laws of genetics and Darwin's theory of evolution.

What is different from those earlier momentous biological discoveries is there is no one individual scientist whose name will become synonymous with the new science of aging. There is no one Ponce de León searching for a fountain of youth. Rather, there has developed a new agglomeration of entities all seeking to lengthen human life, a sort of "aging research–industrial complex." It is a sprawling establishment of government agencies, university departments, foundations, giant corporations, and small biotech startups spending billions of dollars a year on research, transforming what was once the minor medical specialty of gerontology into the dynamic new science of aging. Funding, for the most part, flows from the top down, funneled from the National Institutes of Health and its National Institute of Aging to hundreds of individual scientists and universities, to medical centers and hospitals, to biotech and pharmaceutical firms. Foundations, the health-care industry, and the pharmaceutical and biotechnology industries provide additional funding to their own researchers and to university and medical center scientists in the hopes of furthering their own aging research goals. The results are, like those of most scientific discoveries, usually seemingly mundane bits and pieces of a larger puzzle, occasionally startling and, in the aggregate, dramatically changing the future of all humanity.

It is this host of new information that forms the core of this book and the television series upon which it is based in part. In these pages we shall explore the new science of aging, learn of many of its new discoveries and meet the people who are making them. Here we shall undertake an understanding of the new ideas and techniques in genetics and medicine, in biology and neurochemistry, and in experimental psychology and geriatrics that are blazing the way to a time, perhaps within the next fifty years, when the average life span may well be double what it is today.

The implications of such possibilities strike a note of awe and even a bit of fear even among those doing the research. At a conference held in Los Angeles in March 1999, ten of the foremost scientists working on the problem of extending life met to assess the progress of the last few years. "They were a small group of eminent academic scientists who had their reputations to think of," reported *The New York Times*. "They were repelled by what they saw as the hucksterism and charlatanism that had given attempts to delay human aging a bad name."[1]

Their review of the progress made by scientists around the world in manipulating the life spans of creatures ranging from micro-organisms to people makes even the most outlandish claims of modern-day snake-oil salesmen seem shortsighted. In the laboratory, tiny worms have had their life spans doubled, fruit flies live four times their normal span, and mice and monkeys have had months and years added to what were the presumed limits of their lives.

While the vast majority of the research has been confined

---

1. Kolata, Gina, "Pushing Limits of the Human Life Span," *The New York Times*, March 9, 1999.

to laboratory animals and micro-organisms, a fundamental discovery has emerged. We have learned that the genetic and biochemical pathways that spark and govern all life forms, including our own, are almost identical. "We know we can extend the life span of mammals," said Dr. Judith Campisi, who heads the department of cellular and molecular biology at the Berkeley National Laboratory. "As a result the application of these life-extending technologies we are developing will inevitably be applied to our own lives."

"Given adequate funding, given lucky breaks, how far could we go?" asked Dr. Gregory Stock, the conference organizer, who is director of the program on medicine, technology, and science at the University of California School of Medicine at Los Angeles.

There is still a long way to go with many basic questions still unanswered. But the implications even now are staggering. "It is going to be very hard for us to deal with," Stock said. The idea of expanding the human life span to 150, 200, or more years, "puts a distance between us and all of our history." And it puts humans in uncharted waters. "All of human wisdom on how to live a life," no longer would apply, Stock said.[2]

If the research is in fact realized, the human life span will be 150 or even 200 years of healthy life. The key word here is "healthy," for the goal of all this new aging research is to add not just years to life, but healthy years. As Harvard gerontologist Dr. Thomas Perls points out, "The new paradigm is that aging not necessarily be associated with diseases. There are a number of people out there who demonstrate this idea of

---

2. Kolata, "Pushing Limits of the Human Life Span."

optimal aging, that you can age slowly and avoid diseases associated with aging until the very end of life."

In this book, as in the television series, we meet several of these people who have reached their nineties and even hundreds. Far from the traditional picture of frail and doddering ancients, these are vigorous, healthy, and interesting oldsters. Their zest for life and their humor shine through. From their lives Dr. Perls and other researchers hope to uncover many of the secrets of successful aging. Those secrets, simple rules and ideas really, are immediately and readily applicable to everyone's life.

Among the conclusions already reached by Dr. Perls and many others is the role that genes play in the aging process. These genes, whether in tiny worms, mice, monkeys, or people, are the keys to longevity. A vast amount of research is now devoted to mapping those genes and learning just what happens when they are turned on and off. In a laboratory at the University of Colorado, Dr. Thomas Johnson, a world-famous geneticist, had discovered, in a tiny worm called a nematode, a gene that is responsible for aging. Turn off the gene, and the worms live three times longer than their counterparts with the turned-on gene.

Then there is the work of Dr. Michael Rose. Using the centuries-old techniques of animal husbandry, Rose is breeding a race of long-lived fruit flies. At the Los Angeles conference reported by *The New York Times*, Rose, a professor in the department of ecology and evolutionary biology at the University of California at Irvine, said there was nothing like creating one of these long-lived organisms to make someone a believer. "I've created postponed-aging with my own hands," he said. "I know what it feels like to see one organism on its last legs and another organism that is the same age doing fine."[3]

While geneticists are at the leading edge of aging research, virtually all the biological disciplines are deeply involved. Zoologists are seeking the answers to longevity among different species in the wild. On an island off the coast of Georgia, Steven Austad, professor of zoology at the University of Idaho and a conference attendee, has discovered a population of opossums that have been isolated from the mainland for four thousand years. And these small animals live twice as long as their mainland counterparts. The reason, he found, was a lack of stress, in a sense. With no predators on the island, the pressure of natural selection to reproduce as rapidly as possible and then die a nervous wreck was removed.

"The really fascinating things about these opossums," he concluded, "is that they have changed in a really fundamental way. The genes within each cell of their bodies are operating differently here on the island as a consequence of having lived for generations and generations in this much safer environment."

Another researcher, Dr. Roy Walford, seventy-four, a professor and physician at UCLA, believes diet holds a key to lengthening life. Walford has dramatically extended the lives of laboratory mice and monkeys by a technique known as caloric restriction, a diet low in calories but high in nutrients. "Many people alive today will live not only into the twenty-first century, but beyond it and into the twenty-second century," he declares.

Raj Sohal, a professor of biology at Southern Methodist

---

3. Kolata, "Pushing Limits of the Human Life Span."

University in Dallas, is studying the effects of oxygen free radicals. "Oxygen is a paradoxical substance that we use. On the one hand, it gives us life. It is also very dangerous because its use necessarily involves the generation of radicals, which are slowly killing us. Living and dying are part of the same coin."

By isolating the gene that prevents the formation of free radicals and inserting it into fruit-fly embryos, Sohal has created a superfly that lives more than 30 percent longer than normal flies. "Of course," says Sohal, "the ultimate purpose of our research is to benefit man. Hopefully what we learn would help us understand the basis of the aging process. If we understand the mechanisms of aging, then it is possible that we can come up with some ways to intervene, to ameliorate the effects of aging."

And what is life like for the oldest old? The idea of a frail, doddering old age has been replaced by a vision of health, vigor, and vitality. Miriam Nelson, director of the Center for Physical Activity Programs and Policy at Tufts University's School of Nutrition Science and Policy and an assistant professor of nutrition, shattered an old medical assumption by discovering that age-related muscle loss can be reversed, even for people in their nineties. When she and her colleagues started a strength training and exercise program for elderly women, it was considered risky. But when their research came out, most members of the medical community "were really astounded that these women can rebuild muscle that they have lost as they have gotten older. In just about two months or so, we can see the reversal." Similar results have been found with the aging brain. William Greenough, a neuroscientist at the Beckman Institute for Advanced Science and Technology at the University of Illinois, is finding that old rats' brains become healthier if the rodents are given exercise or taken out of dull lab cages and placed in a stimulating environment.

Exercising the human brain has proven to be just as beneficial. Timothy Salthouse, Regents Professor of Psychology at the Georgia Institute of Technology, is studying the complex everyday skill of typing. Typists, as they age, become slower at striking an individual key. But Salthouse is discovering that older typists can match the number of words per minute of typists half their age. The experience they've gained over the years allows them to read farther ahead and plan the movements of their fingers more efficiently.

What of the loss of mental skills and memory due to such natural events as menopause? Barbara Sherwin, a professor of psychology at McGill University, is finding that the reduction in verbal memory that many women experience at menopause is reversed when they are given estrogen to restore levels that have naturally declined. Hers is the first study to show that a hormone can restore cognitive performance in healthy people.

The loss of mental ability and memory as we age has been one of the most fearful aspects of growing old. But studies have shown this is not necessarily the case for most people. Since 1956, as director of the Seattle Longitudinal Study, K. Warner Schaie has been tracking the mental abilities of a single group of people. The results are defying all expectations. Rather than seeing a steady mental decline over the years, Schaie is discovering that people in their sixties are scoring as high as they did in their twenties.

This and other research, the new knowledge and its implications for the future, are examined in the television series and further amplified in the pages that follow. And where may it all lead? John Rubin, executive producer of the television series, puts it this way: "We can grow in our careers, skills, and passions, even at ages far beyond those we consider for retirement. Aging is an opportunity."

This then is an account of the research and discoveries of the people and places where the newest scientific frontier—the challenge of aging—is being crossed.

1 *The Aging Paradox*

From the moment life begins we are on a journey that inevitably leads to death. For most of human history that journey has been swift, measured in a scant handful of decades. But
now, as we enter the twenty-first century, that relentless journey to decrepitude and ultimate end is being slowed dramatically. More people are living longer than ever before in history.

By the beginning of the twenty-first century more than
fifty-two thousand Americans will be one hundred or more
years old. Only forty years after that, some demographers es-
timate there will be as many as four million Americans one
hundred years or older. Methuselah is no longer a Biblical
myth, but a snowballing demographic reality. Right now the
oldest old, people eighty-five and older, are the fastest growing segment of the population. Between 1960 and 1990, the
overall U.S. population grew 39 percent. But the numbers of
those eighty-five and older exploded exponentially by 232

percent. And this trend is a worldwide phenomenon, re-peated in every other prosperous nation.

Not surprisingly, it is not only senior citizens—the sixties plus generation—that must be concerned with the prospects for vastly increased longevity. The largest group in history to confront the prospect of living to be one hundred are the baby-boomers, the generation now reaching the age of fifty. For several million people now in their forties and fifties, the prospect of reaching one hundred and older is not only a probability, it is inevitable. The implications of this prospect are staggering not only to the individuals concerned, but also to society in general.

Of more concern is the immediate future: will there be legions of doddering, ill, and infirm oldsters overflowing nursing homes, hospitals, and other health-care facilities, be-coming a crushing economic burden on their children, grandchildren, and even great-grandchildren? It is a concept humankind has never before had to confront. The startling gains in medicine, public health, and sanitation over the past century have made a million Methuselahs a reality. But are we in store for an old age Malthusian nightmare? Or is the fu-ture not as grim as it might seem?

"Aging is not a medical condition that needs to be cured," says George Maddox, a professor emeritus at the Duke Aging Center. "Most people associate aging with automatic mental and physical decline, but age is usually not the cause of dis-ability. Disease is the cause of disability, and older people don't have to live with it."[4]

---

4. Levine, Rebecca, "Mapping Aging's Boundaries," *Duke Research,* 1997–98.

"Aging," points out Dr. Thomas Johnson, a geneticist at the Institute of Behavioral Genetics, University of Colorado, "is not programmed. There is not a time bomb that is going off in our cells, that is killing our cells or us. You know we are not programmed to die."

The fact is we stand now on the brink of the day when a newborn can expect to live to the age of 120 and even older, much older.

"Aging is no longer regarded as a monolith, an immovable frontier," states gerontologist Dr. Caleb Finch of the University of Southern California. "We, probably with existing technology, don't have to invent anything new to get to the heart of biological aging. I'm highly optimistic."

But our past experience tells us that life is short and the healthy years even shorter. If we were to graph health across the span of human life it would reach its highest peak at the age of eleven. At that early point in life the aging process has not yet begun. Our bodies glow with vitality, energy, and resilience. If we could but maintain this supreme state of health we could live for a thousand years. But we cannot. We no sooner reach the apex than we begin to decline. The rate varies, but for every human being the onset of adolescence also marks the beginning of aging. Ahead lie the risks of life—pregnancy, the stress of adulthood and parenting, accidents, a decreasing resistance to injury and disease. From that pinnacle of health at the age of eleven, the chance of death doubles every eight years.

Along with the inevitability of death and taxes, the idea of aging as an ever quickening, downhill journey that seemingly gathers speed with each passing day has held the preeminent place in our thinking. But today that belief is being challenged by scientists exploring a new frontier. Now science is questioning why aging, with all its debilitating effects, is even a part of the life process. Why, researchers now ask, if we must die, why must we also decline so abjectly, so pathetically? What is there in the natural scheme of things that forces us into the Shakespearean model from "mewling and puking infant…to…Second childishness, and mere oblivion, sans teeth, sans eyes, sans taste, sans everything?"

One answer is that it has always been so. Aging, debilitation, and disease have been the inevitable human experience. "When I was in medical school we were taught that the older you were the worse off you had to be," remembers Harvard gerontologist Dr. Thomas Perls, author of *Living to 100*. "And certainly a one-hundred-year-old would have to have every disability known under the sun."

Virtually all the old people doctors saw were very ill. It was clinical confirmation of what medical students were being taught. But as an intern, Tom Perls discovered a paradox that challenged the established view of aging. "To my amazement, when I was taking care of a couple of one-hundred-year-olds as a fellow in geriatrics, they were among my healthiest patients. I didn't understand that. That was a true shock to me."

At the time, Perls was a fellow at the Hebrew Home for Aged, one of the Harvard Medical School's geriatric training sites. The young resident was assigned a number of elderly patients, two of whom were actually one hundred years old. Whenever he tried to see them, they were never in their rooms. Perls was puzzled by their absence until he discovered that one was a pianist and every time he tried to look in on her, she was playing the piano for other residents at the center; the other centenarian was a tailor and he was always downstairs sewing people's clothes.

"I actually had to make an appointment to see my patients," he recalls with amusement. It also triggered a consuming curiosity. How did some people seem to escape the degenerative assault of time? Perls had personal experience with the question. On his desk is a picture of himself as a baby, cradled in the arms of his 102-year-old great-grandmother.

In a quest for answers Perls looked to census reports to identify people over one hundred years old. The first surprise was their numbers. They formed a fairly large demographic group. What was even more astonishing they were almost all healthy!

Perls directs the New England Centenarian Study, a population-based survey of all the centenarians in an eight-town area around Boston. Begun in 1995, the study has found that about one of every ten thousand people in the area is a centenarian. Many were in good health and functioning independently, a finding that echoes a national pattern.

"People who make it past eighty-five are a hardy group," says Richard Suzman of the National Institute on Aging. "About 30 percent still live in the community and are robust in the sense that they are able to lift shopping bags, walk half a mile, and climb stairs."

"The really important point about centenarians," emphasizes Perls, "is they are really spending the vast majority of their lives in excellent health.... So we want to find out from these centenarians how they were able to do that."

Among those Perls interviewed was 104-year-old Angeline Strandal of Quincy, Massachusetts. Mrs. Strandal had six brothers and five sisters. Two of her sisters died at the age of one hundred. The others, save for a fourteen-year-old who died of peritonitis, lived into their eighties and nineties. Widowed in 1931, Angeline Strandal still cooks every day but Sunday for her sixty-seven-year-old daughter and a sixty-nine-year-old son. She is blessed with a marvelous sense of humor to complement her good health. Responding to a series of compliments about her general appearance, she said she was not putting on any weight. "I don't want to lose my gorgeous figure."

Perhaps as much as anything, Angeline Strandal has reached 104 because of her attitude. "I don't really feel old at all," she told Tom Perls. "Because oftentimes I will say to people, it's not the figures like 104 or 105, like I am, it is yourself. You can be old, 'oh, I can't get up,' you can say that, but you can get up, see."

In a 1995 report, more than 60 percent of the centenarians followed in another study, the Georgia Centenarian Study, rated their health as good to excellent. "An even higher percentage said it was as good or better than five years ago," notes Martha Bramlett, a project researcher from the Medical College of Georgia. "We know we get a skewed view of the health of centenarians in general because we only look at those who are still community dwelling, but our checkups confirm that they are in remarkably good health. One gentleman, David, who is 105, still reads without glasses and has 20/25 vision. Julia, a retired seamstress, still threads her own needles at one hundred."

Even many of those incapable of living in the community find a way to lead active, rewarding lives in nursing homes and other care facilities. Geneva McDaniel at 105 taught aerobics daily at her senior citizens center. At 107 she led an exercise class of "youngsters" in their eighties and nineties at the nursing home to which she had just moved.

"We can't make generalizations about these very exceptional people because each one is different," says Leonard Poon, Director of the Georgia Centenarian Study. "Centenarians continue to surprise us, so that now, surprises are the rule."

Perls believes centenarians possess some biological ability to resist aging. Gerontologists define the human life span by the oldest member of the species. To date, that record is held by a French woman named Jeanne Calment—the oldest human on record. She lived for 122 years and retained her vitality through her final days. Every day that she lived she extended the presumptive maximum human life span by a day. She aged very slowly and with such amazing prowess Perls dubbed her the "Michael Jordan of aging."

In March 1995, France celebrated Jeanne Calment's 120th birthday, as she became the oldest documented person on earth. "Aging actually suits me rather well," she said marking the occasion. "I had to wait 110 years to become famous and I intend to enjoy it as long as possible."

Among the researchers flocking to Arles to study Madame Calment was Leonard Poon. With him he brought a letter he had asked 107-year-old Mary Sims Elliot to write to Calment. Mrs. Elliot wrote in French, a language she learned more than ninety years ago. When asked how she had remembered French after so many years she replied, "My dear, I learned it very well as a child."

Jeanne Calment eventually died in 1997. She not only had outlived her entire generation and most of those of her children's and grandchildren's generations, but also a man named André-François Raffray. Raffray is an ironic footnote to the remarkable story because thirty-two years before her death, he agreed to pay then ninety-year-old Jeanne Calment $500 a month for the rest of her life in order to purchase her apartment in Arles. Buying apartments, *en viager*, or "for life," as the arrangement is called, is common in France. But on Christmas 1995, Raffray died at the age of seventy-seven, having paid out over $184,000 for an apartment he never got to live in. His widow continued the payments, already far in excess of the apartment's market value. Had she died before Calment passed away in 1997, her children and grandchildren would have had to continue the payments. And that is not beyond the bounds of future probability for the age of 122 is seen as one many centenarians may well surpass with the promising discoveries of the new science of aging.

Researchers draw a sharp distinction between the maximum human life span of 120 years—a figure believed not to have changed since our species evolved—and average longevity, which has increased by leaps and bounds as medicine and hygiene have improved. Consider the remarkable extension of human longevity in just the past century. When today's centenarians were born around 1900, the average human lived for forty-six years. Today, thanks to great advances in public health, vaccines, antibiotics, and other drugs, the average life span has almost doubled to seventy-nine years.

For most of human history, life has been measured out in the most parsimonious of terms. At the time of the Roman Empire the average human life span was eighteen years. In the seventeenth century, life expectancy was under twenty-five years, death was the center of life, and the graveyard the center of every village. For every hundred births there were twenty-five deaths before the age of one year. Another twenty-five died before the age of twenty and still another twenty-five were struck down between the ages of twenty and forty-five. Only ten people out of a hundred ever grew to be sixty. "The triumphant octogenarian," writes historian Pierre Goubert in *Louis XIV and Twenty Million Frenchmen,* "surrounded by an aura of legend that made him seem at least a hundred, was regarded with the superstitious awe spontaneously accorded to champions. His sons and daughters, nephews and nieces long dead, as well as a good half of his grandchildren, the sage lived on to become an oracle for his entire village. His death was a major event for the whole region."

Then in the eighteenth century, infant mortality began to fall. The population, especially of the young, exploded and the rarity of old age began to dim along with the importance of the village elder. At the beginning of the nineteenth century, youth became the focus of society. Young people were perceived as more vital, actually wiser than their curmudgeonly, conservative elders. The modern obsession with looking and being young stems from this crucial cultural shift.

But now we face another cultural shift, the possibility of not just extended life, but extended youth. "People are realizing that life doesn't stop at seventy-five for many of us and that people can expect another ten, fifteen, even twenty years of quality of life ahead of them, and this is an amazing shift for society," says Tom Perls.

It is happening almost by default. Children born today or even the baby-boomers born around 1960 have a far less threatening environment to live in. "So they can fulfill their genetic promise," declares Perls, "if they have the predisposition to get to one hundred, they can get there."

There is more than just a benign environment at work, according to Perls. "One thing is that the baby-boomers, who I now call the elder boomers, are a pretty smart bunch. They pay a lot of attention in general to their nutrition, to exercise. They avoid things like smoking and excess drinking...so they are really putting a lot of things in their favor to maximize their individual life spans."

And as if echoing some enriched variant of Malthusian demographics, it seems that the more centenarians there are, the more there will be. "It really increases peoples' horizons if we know that there are a lot of centenarians out there," says Perls. "I think it increases our own outlook on aging and that it makes us significantly more optimistic about how old we ourselves can get to be."

To Dr. Perls, the really important point about centenarians is that even though some of them, even a substantial number, may have disabilities and other problems at the end of their lives, all of them were in excellent health well into their early to mid-nineties. "They are really spending the vast majority of their lives in excellent health and certainly if all of us could do that that would be fantastic," he says.

It is this idea of a healthy life virtually to the end of life that has led doctors to a new paradigm of aging. "The new paradigm," explains Perls, "is that aging not necessarily be associated with diseases. There are a number of people out there who demonstrate this idea of optimal aging, that you can age slowly and avoid diseases associated with aging until the very end of life."

Doctors call it the compression of morbidity. "You live the vast majority of life in excellent health only to have the very last bit spent with diseases," says Perls. "So we want to find out from these centenarians how they were able to do that, and we know that involves aging extremely slowly and also having a decreased susceptibility to diseases associated with aging and probably depending upon what combination of genes you have, how well you avoid things that we know are hazardous to people's health."

Among centenarians, good health, Dr. Perls discovered, is the norm rather than the exception. They are healthier as a group than the merely elderly. The biggest killers, heart disease and stroke, for example, have their greatest impact on men in their fifties through eighties. For women those killers hit about ten years later. Once past a certain age, the fatal risk of those diseases is reduced dramatically. Other crippling diseases of the elderly, such as Alzheimer's disease, arc also a minor factor. Indeed, studies have found that men in their nineties do better on tests of mental function than do octogenarians. Even death itself takes a bit of holiday among centenarians. For while the risk of dying rises exponentially each year from fifty to ninety, it slows appreciably after age ninety.

And the cost of dying goes down as we get older. As cited in the Introduction, a 1995 study by the Health Care Financing Administration calculated that medical expenditures for the last two years of life average $22,600 for people who die at seventy, but just $8,300 for those who live to be one hundred.

The cost of caring for the elderly is also heading down. The Duke University Center for Demographic Studies examined the results of the National Long-Term Care Surveys of the nation's elderly populations sponsored by the National Institute on Aging. The Duke researchers found that from 1982 to 1994 the chronic disability rates for people sixty-five and older in the United States decreased almost 15 percent. "If the rates had held steady from 1982 to 1994, there would be 1.2 million more older people with chronic disabilities in the United States than there actually are," said Duke demographer Kenneth Manton. "There were about 7.1 million chronically disabled people in the nation in 1994. Disability declines of this size may have important implications for national health-care costs. For example, the 1994 United States institutional population was estimated to be 1.7 million persons. The 1982 rates, after age standardization, implied 2.1 million persons would be institutionalized in 1994. The difference of 400,000 implies, assuming an annual per capita nursing home cost in 1994 of $43,300, savings of $17.3 billion in nursing home expenses in 1994."

The cost of medical care will drop even further as the baby-boom generation grows old. The net result will be to ease pressure on Medicare and the fears that it will go bankrupt under the weight of an avalanche of claims from hordes of sick and infirm, aging baby-boomers. In fact, a study co-authored by H. Dennis Tolley, a professor of statistics at Brigham Young University, and six other researchers suggested that improved medical technology could eventually lower total health-care costs and even boost the economy. "Most people become eligible for Medicare when they turn sixty-five," explains Tolley. "From that point, a person who lives to be ninety will incur less overall health-care costs than a person who lives to be seventy-five, even though the first person lived fifteen years longer," reports Tolley.

The probable reason for this unlikely circumstance is that lower health maintenance costs for older people may be due to their avoiding the early risk of many chronic diseases. But it is the seemingly illogical idea that health care of the elderly will be a boon rather than a drain on the economy that is surprising. The traditional outlook is that the increasing cost of new technology absorbs any savings resulting from better health. "When technologies for a particular disease are in their intermediate stage of development, they often do cost more than traditional treatments," says Tolley. "But once technologies reach an advanced stage, they save money. Look at cataract surgery—nowadays it's no big deal, but back in 1970 it was so serious they had to sandbag your head for a week."

Based on their research, Tolley and his colleagues suggest worries about Medicare's future may be overblown. For example, official predictions don't take into account the improving health of the elderly population. "Medicare predictions take recent years' costs and project them over the next ten years," he notes. "But right now we are in an era where the maximum number of ex-smokers are turning sixty-five and entering Medicare eligibility. That number will go down as generations more attendant to their health enter the Medicare-age bracket." A healthier population will miss less time from work and need less attention from family caretakers, thus boosting worker productivity, the authors say.[5]

The reason for this sudden spurt in healthiness is in part a product of natural selection. "The genetically weak die off," points out Perls. "What is left is an enriched group of healthy, strong individuals." But, genetics are not the only component of successful aging. A lifestyle of moderation, exercise, and education also pays off, according to Perls. Vigorous and healthy, these are not ancient fossils to be warehoused

---

5. "Dying Older Is Cheaper," *Brigham Young University Report*, January 6, 1999.

in nursing homes, shunted out of the mainstream of American life. About 15 percent of all centenarians live by themselves. Another 35 percent live with a family member and 50 percent are in nursing homes.

After interviewing one hundred centenarians Perls has discovered they share intriguing similarities. Centenarians are unlikely to die of cancer. Women are more likely to have had children late in life—a sign of slow aging. Most centenarians have relatives who have also reached one hundred—a sign they may inherit some ability to remain healthy as they get older.

Perls has uncovered a great deal of evidence to support this idea. "We have located a number of families that have a lot of family members who reach very old age. One family we discovered from Ohio had three centenarians and a person in their nineties all in the same generation. All brothers and sisters."

Ironically those families are studied statistically as if they had a genetic disease running through them. "You want to study the family looking for genes that predispose that family to the disease," explains Perls. "In this instance, it's not a disease, it's the ability to live to a very old age." Perls turned up another form of evidence in the family trees of 102 centenarians. They all had brothers and sisters at an increased chance of reaching a very old age themselves. For Tom Perls, the real challenge in the future will be to try and identify those genes associated with the aging process and use that to learn how the rest of us can maximize our own life expectancies.

Advances in sanitation, medicine, and other improvements have, as we've seen, almost doubled the average human life expectancy in this century alone. But that still leaves us far short of the presumed 115-year built-in capacity of our genes or the 122 years achieved by Jeanne Calment. Eating right, exercising, taking vitamins, and doing all the other good stuff we hear about might buy us a few more years but that still leaves us far short of the 120- to 150-year life span most gerontologists believe is achievable. Even those seemingly remarkable ages may not be the ultimate limit.

For the last hundred years, the maximum life span of many species, including humans, was based upon the so-called Gompertz Mortality Model. Using the model, developed by Benjamin Gompertz, a nineteenth-century British actuary, demographers and others have calculated that the rate of human mortality doubles every eight years after puberty. But a mathematical analysis of the Gompertz model by Dr. Caleb Finch and colleague Dr. Malcom C. Pike factors in the mortality of centenarians. At 100 or 105, for example, the rate of acceleration slows down dramatically. The result is the possibility that humans might live longer in the future than anyone has ever imagined.

"We've thought there was a maximum age beyond which no one could live," notes John Wilmoth, an assistant professor of demography at the University of California, Berkeley, Center for the Economics and Demography of Aging, "but I think that's a common myth. So far, we've seen a continuous rise in achieved age. I don't think we can live forever, but we haven't yet been able to find a fixed limit for the human life span. Consistent with this upward trend in longevity, increasing numbers of people are living to be one hundred years old."

Wilmoth detected an increase in the maximum longevity of particular national populations, suggesting that the upper limit on the human life span is slowly rising over time by about one year for every two decades. In Sweden, which has kept the best records in the world, there has been a remarkably steady trend upward in the maximum age achieved by the elderly population over a period of 130 years, according to Wilmoth.

"We think that it probably doesn't take anything special from a genetic point of view to live to an average life expectancy age seventy-five," says Tom Perls. "But to get to one hundred, I think another twenty-five years of a person's life really takes some very special talent, and that talent is probably in the form of genes."

Genes, of course, determine far more than physical shape, hair, and eye color. Genes operate on the cellular level instructing the various organelles in the cells to make enzymes, various proteins, and hormones, to divide and to stop dividing, and complete a host of other duties that determine the body's ability to grow, fight off disease, and repair itself.

With each new discovery, it becomes increasingly apparent that nature has engineered the body to last far longer than it does. This phenomenon lies in evolution. Nature selects for the survival of the species, not the individual. The cells that comprise any organism are designed as the carriers of the species' survival in the form of genes. The passage of those genes from one generation to the next is the ultimate goal of all life. "A chicken is an egg's way of making another egg" is one of the more whimsical metaphors biologists use to describe this idea.

Reproduction then is guaranteed by enabling the cells to live long enough to pass on their genes. Factored into the mix are allowances for individual losses to predation and disease. Nature then adds a safety margin, in the form of cellular repair kits, guaranteeing enough organisms will live long enough to pass their genes on to the next generation.

As a result, from an evolutionary viewpoint, long life makes no sense because most creatures are either eaten, struck by a virus, or hit by a truck. Nature therefore has selected those genes that promote quick and prolific breeding over those that favor long life.

British biologist Thomas Kirkwood of the University of Manchester calls this the "disposable soma" theory. "Soma" is Latin for body, and so we may also think of it as nature's version of a throwaway body. The idea is that aging is a product of accumulated unrepaired defects in body cells. The genes that are programmed to repair those cells and are thus the primary genetic controllers of longevity have been forced by natural selection to raise or lower the investment in basic cellular maintenance systems in relation to the level of environmental hazard the organism faces.

The idea of reproduction as life's highest calling seems to hold true for all life forms. In most species, nature seems to favor the female. "We have noticed for quite some time now that when we go and see centenarians more than likely it is going to be a woman on the other side of the door," remarks Dr. Thomas Perls. "In fact about 90 percent of centenarians are women. So we know that women have the edge in terms of being able to achieve extreme age, and we are trying now to discover why that is. We think that from an evolutionary point of view the idea is to have as many young as you can have to pass your genes down to subsequent generations. In order to do that, certainly you would want to age as slowly as possible so that you can extend the period of time during which you can have children."

As a consequence, our extended lives often bring about some rather unwelcome consequences. It's a sort of evolutionary trade-off—heightened reproductive powers early in life and increasing mortality later. "The essence of the idea, which has acquired the forbidding label 'negative pleiotropy,'[6] is that genes have evolved that confer marked advantages on an organism at certain stages in its life, only to extract a cost at certain other stages," indicates Robert Sapolsky, an assistant professor of biology and neuroscience at Stanford University.

Sapolsky calls these genes double-edged swords. He offers sickle cell anemia as an example of such negative pleiotropy. The gene causes a life-threatening disease by preventing hemoglobin from delivering sufficient oxygen to the cells. Yet that same gene confers an immunity to malaria, a killer disease that ravaged Africa for millennia.

But where aging is considered negative pleiotropy over time, sickle cell anemia, Sapolsky points out, might more properly be thought of as negative pleiotropy over space, offering benefits only where malaria is endemic. "In the evolution of such trade-offs," Sapolsky informs us, "the critical issue becomes how often the advantage is conferred compared with how often the deleterious bill arrives. Apparently, with sickle cell anemia the payoffs have led to widespread selection for the trait. That is small comfort to sickle cell victims who live in, say, urban America where shored up resistance to malaria is of little use. Betrayed by geography, American carriers of the sickle cell gene are forced to pay its price without enjoying any of its benefits."[7]

---

6. In genetics, pleiotropy is the ability of a gene to manifest or express itself in several ways.

7. Sapolsky, Robert M., and Finch, Caleb E., "On Growing Old," *The Sciences*, April/May 1991.

For most creatures longevity is made possible by the ability of the body to repair itself. "We tend to think of ourselves and other animals in the same way we think of machines: wearing out is inevitable," declares Steven Austad, a professor of zoology at the University of Idaho. "Yet biological organisms are fundamentally different from machines. They are self-repairing: wounds heal, bones mend, illness passes. Why then should they be subject to the same sorts of wear and tear as machines?"

In fact, they are not. Aging is far more than a simple process of decay, of wearing away. The human body is a work in progress, under constant repair. Even when we sleep, our cuts and bruises heal. The cells and molecules in our body are being replaced. Fresh layers of skin protect us from the world around us. The person we see in the mirror looks the same as it did a month ago, but many of the molecules that comprise our body are new. And the process continues throughout life, but with diminishing efficiency. For biologists the degree of self-repair determines the rate at which we age.

The process is akin to deciding how long to keep a car in good repair. Like our bodies, our cars must be maintained and repaired. When accidents take their toll, we knock out the dents, sand, and repaint. If we had the money, we could keep our cars running forever. But at some point it makes sense to cut back on repairs and save up for a new car.

"Aging," says Dr. Jared Diamond, a physiologist at the UCLA School of Medicine, "is a failure of self-repair. We are constantly repairing our bodies. The most familiar example is our skin. If you cut your skin, a scar forms and your skin heals over. Or, for instance, we repair our teeth. Once in our lifetime our baby teeth fall out and we grow adult teeth.

Now elephants do better, they replace their teeth five times. Sharks replace their teeth an infinite number of times. So aging is a matter of self-repair."

Different species, even those whose genetic heritage is identical, age at different rates. "Our closest relatives," points out Diamond, "are the African great apes, chimpanzees, and gorillas. We are astonishingly close to them. It's been realized in the last decade or so that we share 98.5 percent of our genes with chimpanzees and 98.2 percent with gorillas. So we are slightly modified chimpanzees and gorillas. And yet you put a chimpanzee in a zoo and give a chimpanzee the best medical care and diet possible and the best safety—chimps in zoos live more pampered lives than the vast majority of Americans—and yet zoo chimps are almost all dead before their late fifties. Whereas an American, given a marginal diet, car accidents, and bad medical care, still has an average life span into his or her early eighties. So there has been a slow down in the aging of humans in the five million years since we diverged evolutionarily from the chimpanzees."

Why should this be so? "Our slow aging means that we put more biological energy into repairing ourselves then a chimpanzee does," answers Diamond. "And we put a lot more energy into it than a mouse does, but we devote less to repair than does an albatross or a tortoise. You can then ask, why is it worth more to repair a human than a chimpanzee and worth less to repair a human than an albatross? That then is another piece of the puzzle."

At first glance it would seem the chimpanzee has all the advantages. About the same size as a human, chimps are far stronger, faster, and possessed of finely honed survival skills, including the ability to flee into the trees from danger.

Moreover, chimps and other great apes use sticks and make other crude tools to aid in food gathering. "But," notes Diamond, "chimpanzees do not make spears and bows and arrows. So a chimpanzee and a gorilla are much more at risk of being killed by leopards and lions than are humans. It means that, apart from aging, a human is more likely to survive accidents and attacks by big predators than a chimpanzee. Therefore it is more worth while to repair a human then it is to repair a chimpanzee. Because if a human takes good care of himself or herself, that human is likely to escape the leopards and lions until even into his or her eighties. Whereas a chimpanzee is unlikely, very unlikely, to escape the leopards or lions beyond its fifties."

The answer perhaps lies in the distinctive lifestyle changes made by humans and their direct ancestors since diverging more than five million years ago from the evolutionary track taken by other primates. Humans developed sophisticated tools and social skills to aid in the hunt and to better protect themselves from the other predators that were individually so much stronger than they were. To learn these skills, human children required far more care for longer periods of time than other primates, providing another imperative to lengthen human life. Only if the parents survived long enough to hand down the accumulated wisdom of survival could reproduction of the next generation be assured.

Nature provided the way by increasing the human life span, but not the reproductive life of women. It shuts down in mid-life. This mechanism is called menopause and it is unique to humans, killer whales, and pilot whales. These creatures are social animals that live and hunt in large groups. Like children, killer whale and pilot whale calves depend on their mothers for many years—a behavior that may explain the paradox of menopause.

All women are born with a finite amount of eggs; men on the other hand retain the ability to produce new sperm continuously. With both partners needed to make babies, why then limit menopause to women? One answer is that childbirth is inherently dangerous. By shutting down a woman's reproductive ability, menopause dramatically improves the chances of her being able to raise her existing children to adulthood.

"Menopause evolved in women and not in men because women are at risk of dying in childbirth," says Jared Diamond. "In the good old days before modern medicine and obstetric care, which is to say until one hundred years ago, death in childbirth was a big risk for women. After all the human baby at birth weighs about six pounds and the average woman is 120 pounds. The infant gorilla at birth weighs three pounds and the mother gorilla is two hundred pounds. I never heard of a mother gorilla or chimpanzee dying in childbirth, but because the human infant is so large, death in childbirth is a big risk and that risk began to be minimized only a century ago."

Still, menopause is almost a contradiction because it shuts down the ability to pass on genes while allowing life to continue. "Menopause," says Diamond, "is really bizarre because natural selection favors those things that pass on our genes. Here natural selection has led to something that forbids a woman from passing on her genes anymore. You would think that a gene for menopause would be the first thing that natural selection ought to eliminate. So why on earth did natural selection permit this paradoxical trait to evolve?"

Primarily because human children have a lot more to

learn than their closest genetic cousins, the great apes. "The human child is dependent on its parents for far longer than the offspring of any other animal," points out Diamond. "Once it is weaned, once it is no longer taking its mother's milk, the mother sits it down next to some leaves or fruit tree and the baby chimpanzee reaches out and grabs the leaves and feeds itself."

Human children face a far more daunting task and the ability to feed oneself requires specialized knowledge, tools, and skills that can take almost two decades to acquire. The loss of parents during that period is a disaster. In traditional societies even orphaned children who had almost reached their teens were likely to die from lack of care.

"Even today," says Diamond, "it is difficult for a single mother. Therefore when a woman dies in childbirth, not only is her fetus dying, but she is jeopardizing the lives of all her previous children. So the older a women gets, the more investment she is putting at risk with every new childbirth. The older she gets, the more likely she is to die in childbirth and the more likely any fetus is to have a genetic malformation anyway."

That, according to Diamond, would have been a big evolutionary mistake. "She should have undergone menopause, forgot that last baby and just been conservative and insured the survival of her previous four babies."

The idea is controversial. Most prehistoric women never made it past the age of thirty, much less to fifty or so, when the hot flashes kick in. Menopause then, says one group of biologists, is nothing more than a technological artifact, with sanitation, medicine, and an absence of predators combining to allow women to live longer than their egg supply.

"For most of our existence we simply didn't live that long," said Dr. Alison Galloway, an anthropologist at the University of California at Santa Cruz. "Menopause happens because through technology we've extended our lives to the point where we run out of egg follicles. There's nothing beneficial about it."[8]

Other researchers, however, point out that a woman's ovaries do not shut down at age thirty or so, but instead they last for forty or forty-five years, the same length of time as our close genetic cousins, chimps and gorillas. More than a handful of hardy stone-age women lived much longer than the average thirty-year-old of her time and thereby lived past the age of menopause. And that may have played a major role in the survival of their families and ultimately the human species.

"Only with the ascent of the grandmother," says Dr. Kristen Hawkes of the University of Utah, "were human ancestors freed to exploit new habitats, to go where no other hominid or primate had gone before.... The grandmother hypothesis gives us a whole new way of understanding why modern humans suddenly were able to go everywhere and do everything. It may explain why we took over the planet."[9]

Jared Diamond saw stark evidence of the role of the grandmother in his studies of preliterate tribes in New Guinea only recently thrust into the modern world. "In New Guinea," he explains, "most people die before they are fifty or fifty-five, but some people live into their eighties or even early nineties. These people who are eighty years old, may be blind, unable

---

8. Angier, Natalie, "Theorists See Evolutionary Advantages in Menopause," *The New York Times,* September 16, 1997.

9. Angier, "Theorists See Evolutionary Advantages in Menopause."

to walk, they may have lost all their teeth, but they are regarded as so precious by the rest of society that their friends and relatives go to great efforts to keep them alive. One thing that is standard in New Guinea is to see an old person who has lost all his teeth so he can't chew. So their relatives chew for him...sweet potatoes or meat and then spit it out into a cup, the soft stuff, the mush, and then the old person can take in the mush and swallow it without chewing."

Diamond sees a stark contrast between the treatment of the elderly in New Guinea and in the United States, Europe, and much of the industrial world. "The basic problem," he says, "is that old people have lost all of their distinctive function in society and the result is they are not valued. They may still be loved, if they have had good relationships with their friends and relatives, but someone in their eighties and nineties is, in general, not the underpinnings of society. In New Guinea it is the reverse. Remember that there was no writing in New Guinea, there was no literacy until the arrival of Europeans. Without writing the repositories of information are the memories of people, especially the memories of old people. So the old people are the encyclopedias. They are incredibly important."

While doing field studies on Reynold Island, Diamond asked people what fruits they ate. There are three types of fruit, he was told. There were wild fruits that were eaten all the time, and there were fruits that were never eaten because they were poisonous or bad tasting. And then there were fruits that were eaten at the time of Hunga Kenga.

The Hunga Kenga, Diamond learned, was a cyclone that had smashed into the island sixty-six years before. It had knocked down the forest and destroyed the gardens. People were forced to forage for whatever they could find, eating foods that they would not normally eat.

How, Diamond wondered, did these people know at the time of the Hunga Kenga what foods normally uneaten were in fact edible? He found the answer in the memories of an old woman, who could only sit in front of her hut, her eyes filmed over by cataracts, her only food the mush from a chewing cup. She had been a young girl, not quite of marriageable age, perhaps ten years old when that cyclone hit in 1900. When another cyclone hit the island some years later, the woman's memories of what was edible meant survival for her village.

"She meant the difference between everybody starving to death and people knowing what fruits they could safely eat," says Diamond. "That really brought home to me the value of old people as the encyclopedia of a preliterate society."

The older a woman is when she first gives birth seems to be at least, in part, a predictor of long life. A study of roughly 1200 years of the British aristocracy's genealogical records found that long-lived married women tended to have later first births and fewer children than other women.

Some researchers put it down to the physical toll exacted by giving birth and raising a family that shortens a woman's life span. It could also be argued that life in drafty castles without plumbing or central heating can be a drag on longevity.

An idea that is gaining increasing currency among many researchers goes to the heart of the role of natural selection on longevity. There is, they claim, a genetic trade-off between fertility and longevity in women. Those who are genetically programmed for long life are less fertile.

"If you have to invest such an enormous amount of energy

into maintaining the body for a long life, there must be a cost," says Rudi G.J. Westendorp of Leiden University Medical Center in Leiden, the Netherlands. "And the theory says there's a cost in fertility."

Westendorp and the co-author of the study, Thomas B. L. Kirkwood of the University of Manchester in England, studied the computerized records of 13,667 married women aristocrats born in Britain between the years 740 and 1875.

Women who died between age fifty and eighty had an average of 2.4 to 2.6 children each, while those who lived into their eighties averaged 2.1 children. Those who reached their nineties had only an average of 1.8 offspring.

The researchers also found a link between life span and a woman's age when she gave birth to her first child. Those who died between ages fifty and eighty gave birth to their first child on average at age 24.3. By contrast, women who lived into their eighties had their first child just past the age of twenty-five. The ninety-year-olds did not give birth to a first child until an average age of twenty-seven.[10]

Dr. Thomas Perls also sees the heavy hand of natural selection behind older women and first-time births and longevity. In a study of centenarian women, Perls and his colleagues at the Harvard Medical School found them much more likely to have had children in middle age than a comparable group of women who died at age seventy-three. Comparing the two groups, born in 1896, who were equivalent in race, religion, and other factors, Perls found that of the fifty-four women who died in 1969 at age seventy-three, only

---

10. "Research Links Low Fertility, Long Life in Females," The Associated Press, December 24, 1998.

5.5 percent had given birth in their forties. Among the centenarians, a whopping 19.5 percent had children after forty, one woman at age fifty-three.

All of the children born to both groups were the product of natural reproduction unaided by fertility enhancing techniques. The dramatic difference in maternal ages is, according to the researchers, clear evidence of natural selection at work. They concluded the genes that kept the centenarians fruitful for so long continued working overtime, long after menopause, to extend the women's lives—evidence that a mother's extended survival is essential to her children's survival.

For more than five million years, that pattern has been shaped by the force of natural selection on our genes. And, as we shall see, natural selection has favored the longevity of humankind over almost all other species.

2   *Other Species*

Compared with most mammals, human beings are virtual Methuselahs. The laboratory rat, for example, despite a total absence of predators, a perfect diet, and the best of care, has become a doddering ancient at the age of two, plagued by cataracts, reproductive problems, and memory loss. Death soon follows. The pattern holds for most living things; only the rate varies. Mice may live to the age of four, dogs to fifteen, horses and chimpanzees to forty. African elephants have life spans of seventy years. And human beings by adding health foods, vitamins, antibiotics, transplants, and step aerobics have managed to place one or two individuals at the 120-year mark. The conclusion one might draw is, for mammals at any rate, bigger is better.

The idea was incorporated in a theory devised by German physiologist Max Rubner that pound for pound all mammals expended the same amount of energy during their lifetimes. In 1884 Rubner demonstrated that no one particular type of food produced energy. The body used carbohydrates, fats, and proteins with equal readiness. In 1894 he proved that the energy produced by the body from food was exactly the same in quantity as it would have been if those same foods were burned in a fire. This meant the laws of thermodynamics governed living tissues as well as the inanimate world. It also upset a widely held theory called vitalism, which posited that there was one set of natural laws for living tissue and another for inanimate material.

Building on these experiments, Rubner then discovered a relationship between metabolic rate (the speed at which the body burns energy), body size, and longevity. His conclusion was that the faster the energy is consumed, the shorter the life, or conversely, the slower the rate, the longer the life. Rubner went on to measure precisely the metabolic rate of five species he could easily observe: guinea pigs, cats, dogs, cows, and horses. Although the size of the animals varied enormously—from the one-pound guinea pig to the thousand-pound horse—with very different life spans—six years for the guinea pig and fifty years for the horse—to Rubner, the conclusion was obvious: metabolic rate determined life span. Metabolic rate is a measure of biochemical activity within the cell, and virtually all mammalian cells are the same size. Rubner found that guinea pigs burned about 260 calories per gram of body weight while horses burned about 170 calories per gram. (When Rubner did his studies, horses were thought to live only thirty years. Based on the newer measure of a fifty-year life span, the horse's metabolic rate is 280 calories, bringing it much closer to that of the guinea pig's 260 calories.)

Rubner's work was popularized as the "rate of living theory" some twenty years later by Raymond Pearl, a biologist at Johns Hopkins University. Pearl was so convinced that aging could be explained as the inevitable by-product of the metabolic rate, he wrote an article in 1927 for *The Baltimore Sun* entitled "Why Lazy People Live the Longest."

Pearl also believed that aging affected the ability to think rationally and advocated the placement of an upper limit of fifty on the voting age. Pearl was obviously not a card-carrying member of the America Association of Retired Persons. Nonetheless, the rate of living theory gained a great deal of scientific credibility and adherents, and there reached a point where predicted life spans were being measured in the amount of oxygen consumed, breaths taken, and heart beats expended. Mice were clocked at a billion heartbeats over their three-and-a-half-year life span, while elephant's hearts were found to thump the same number of times over the course of a seventy-year life. But the theory unglues on the human heart, which trip-hammers away at three billion times during a seventy-five-year span.

Despite the anomaly of the human heart beating three times longer than any other mammalian species, some very recent research in a narrow mathematical discipline called scaling seemingly lends credence to the relationship between size and heart rate. Scaling measures the relationship of phenomena such as heart rate to body size according to a precise mathematical principle called quarter-power scaling. The cat, which is one hundred times larger than a mouse, lives approximately three times longer, or one hundred to the one-quarter power.[11] The cat's heart in life, and according to formula, thus beats a third as fast as a mouse.

The application of scaling theory to such biological phenomena as heart rate and life span is the product of an interdisciplinary collaboration between two biologists and a physicist. Geoffrey West, a theoretical high-energy physicist at the U.S. Department of Energy's Los Alamos National Laboratory, and biologists James Brown of the University of New Mexico and Brian Enquist of the Santa Fe Institute joined forces at the Santa Fe Institute, an interdisciplinary research center in New Mexico. Their goal was to apply scaling to explain the subtle ways in which various characteristics of living creatures—their life spans, their pulse rates, how fast they burn energy—change according to their body size.

"Life is the most complex physical system in the universe," says West. "Beyond natural selection, genetic codes, and the like, there are hardly any general principles or laws that we know that it obeys. Scaling laws are the exception. These are quantitative laws and, remarkably, they are absurdly simple given you are dealing with the most complex of systems."

West, Brown, and Enquist base their model on the idea that a common mechanism underlies life—the way materials are transported through the linear networks that supply all parts of an organism. These transport systems, in reality the pipes through which fluids flow, whether mammalian

---

11. If you have a calculator with a square root sign take the square root of 100, which is 10, and then take the square root of 10, which is 3.2. The heartbeat scales to mass, to the **minus** one-quarter power.

blood vessels or plant vascular systems, are, in turn, based on three unifying principles.

First, for the network to supply the entire organism the network system must fill the entire space by branching into every part. Second, the final branch of the network, such as a capillary in the circulatory system, must be the same size in every organism. For example, the capillary in a mouse is the same size as that in a lion. Finally, the energy required to distribute resources throughout the organism is reduced to the minimal amount of energy required to keep it alive.

The result is an exquisite mechanism that keeps the metabolic rate in tune with the size of the animal and measures out its life in direct relation to its size.

Although the rate of living theory influenced gerontological thinking for many years, it just does not hold up in the light of present day knowledge. "We have no evidence, even anecdotal," wrote Dr. Leonard Hayflick, a professor of anatomy at the University California, San Francisco, in his book *How and Why We Age*,[12] "that the aging process is accelerated in people or animals whose rate of living or energy expenditure is high, no matter how the theory is defined."

No matter the cause, inevitably, most creatures age as they grow older, they sicken, and they die. For some living things, however, growing older does not mean an inevitable decline. "In terms of evolution," declares Whitfield Gibbons, a professor of ecology at the University of Georgia's Savannah River Ecology Laboratory, "the measure of success is passing genes on to the next generation, not how long you live."

---

12. Hayflick, Leonard, *How and Why We Age*, Ballantine Books, New York, 1994, p. 241.

Gibbons works in the lab's three hundred square miles of forest and wetland along the Savannah River in the heart of South Carolina. The laboratory was founded in 1951 with a modest grant from what was then known as the Atomic Energy Commission, which was planning to build a reactor to produce plutonium for nuclear weapons on the site. The AEC wanted to inventory the local plants and animals in the area before the reactors were built in order to assess the environmental effects once the plant was in operation. They turned to Eugene Odum, then an associate professor of biology at the University of Georgia. Odum asked for a grant of $150,000, which the AEC immediately rejected. His next request was perhaps the biggest bargain in the history of ecological science—$11,934. Broken down his budget called for $2200 each for three graduate students, $1750 for a pickup truck, $1700 for field expenses, $1000 for field equipment and supplies, and $884 for overhead. The university offered to throw in support for two senior researchers, secretarial assistance, and a reference collection and library.

It was an offer the AEC could not refuse, and on June 23, 1951, the first researchers were in the field. In 1964, the laboratory finally was given an official name and in 1972 was designated the nation's first National Environmental Research Park. It is off-limits to the public and its flora and fauna as well as the scientists who work there are undisturbed by tourists.

In this pristine natural environment Whit Gibbons has been trapping and studying turtles since 1967. Over the years he and his colleagues have captured and recaptured almost twenty thousand animals to learn how they endure over time.

Turtles are among the longest-lived reptiles. "Turtles definitely live longer than dogs, horses, and deer," says Gibbons, "because many species of turtles have been documented now to live more than thirty years. But the question is, when do they stop living? There are records, documented records of turtles over seventy-five years old."

In fact, the champion senior citizen among turtles was a giant tortoise that resolutely plodded among the cannons of a British fortress on the island of Mauritius for 150 years. Captured in 1768, the lumbering giant lived a sprightly and, for a turtle, dignified existence. But, in 1918, the huge tortoise got too close to the edge, fell through a gun port, and died. Were it not for its Humpty Dumpty ending, the giant reptile might have set a longevity record for sentient creatures. For turtles, as Gibbons and other scientists have learned, may get old, but they don't seem to die of old age.

"I'm definitely aging faster than the turtles I'm catching," acknowledges Gibbons. "Sure, they're getting older and I'm getting older at the same rate. But they're not showing it nearly as much as I am. They aren't showing a lot of the traits that humans show: we don't see osteoporosis in turtles; we don't see them getting cataracts; we don't see their eyesight getting weaker. An older turtle is just older, and they probably get wiser, but they don't show the aging that we do as humans. If you look at an individual that looked old twenty years before, thirty years before, it doesn't look any older today—it is older but it hasn't aged. And when it's a female it's still laying eggs; if it's a male it's still mating every year. So they continue with no evidence of major physiological changes like we're seeing in humans. They get older, but they don't age."

Gibbons determines the age of young turtles by counting the growth rings on the shell, much like a forester dates a tree. When they are recaptured, it is a simple matter to count the new rings and add them to the number of years since the first capture. The trick is to be able to identify individual turtles. Gibbons does that by using another feature of the turtle's anatomy, the twenty-four or so plates (the number varies slightly between species) that comprise the shell. He has devised a code that not only determines who each individual is, sort of a Social Security number, but also identifies where and when it was first captured and marked.

As a back-up the smaller, captured turtles are also photocopied. The young turtles will grow, get larger, but they will still look the same, with the same patterns on the shell, the same configuration, and the same number of plates.

Finally the female turtles are x-rayed to count their eggs. The x-rays, according to Gibbons, are very important for these kinds of ecological studies. "We want to keep all of our animals alive, especially in terms of the aging studies. The old-fashioned way of determining how many eggs are in a turtle, snake, or lizard was to cut them open. You do that and that's the last time you're going to learn anything about that individual. The x-rays allow us to determine how many eggs that individual has and because it is nondestructive, it allows us to tell how many eggs that individual has next year, ten years from now, and twenty years from now. So it allows us to get cumulative information on individuals."

This cumulative information provides the most telling evidence that turtles do not age as they grow old. "The number of eggs a turtle lays is not likely to decrease over time," explains Gibbons, "which you'd expect if they were really showing an aging process like many animals do. Humans, for example, become less reproductive as they get older. Turtles, if anything, become more reproductive because as they get older and bigger, they generally lay more eggs. A female turtle that started laying eggs when she was eight to ten years old, if she lives to be seventy years old, she's going to still be laying eggs every year. If it's a male it's still mating every year."

Most species of turtles continue to do this for thirty or forty years. "In contrast to humans," says Gibbons, "a five-decade-old mud turtle would probably look and behave just like one half its age." It's a remarkable achievement considering the hazards a turtle must face from the moment its mother scrapes a hole in the sand, drops in a clutch of eggs, and waddles unconcernedly away. "Think what survivors they are," marvels Gibbons. "They're on their own from the time they hatch out of that egg. For the next thirty or forty years they have to face different weather conditions and predators and they do that very well."

Indeed, the risk of adult turtles dying prematurely in the wild is very low. Gibbons and his colleagues have found that for ten-year-old mud turtles, almost ninety out of every hundred reach the age of eleven. That same turtle at the age of twenty-five has the same chance of reaching the age of twenty-six.

What confers these remarkable survival skills upon the turtle? The turtle has had 200 million years to perfect a genetic plan that provides it with a virtually impenetrable armor against the hazards of the environment: its shell. "The shell," explains Gibbons, "insulates its owner against a wide range of temperatures and moisture conditions and, more important, deters most potential enemies. Foxes, opossums, and most other terrestrial predators are likely to lose interest in a meal shut up inside a container that can't be opened. Aquatic predators are also likely to seek more tractable prey than an armored tank that has sharp claws and a biting mouth."

For turtles, natural selection has obviously chosen the armor-plated shell as the ideal genetic plan for longevity. Nature has other long-term survival plans for other classes of animals. Wings offer escape from earth-bound predators. As a result, birds live three times longer than mammals of similar size. Large size is another form of protection. Elephants are among the most long-lived mammals on earth. For others there is camouflage. Lions and tigers blend in with their backgrounds to conceal them from prey and make them successful hunters. Some insects resemble sticks or leaves to confuse predators. Others adopt the coloration of those that are poisonous, and others simply don't taste very good.

Safer environments make some animals extremely long-lived. Queen bees may live from five to fifteen years, while worker bees even with the same genetic structure may not last a year. The difference is the environment—queens lead pampered and protected lives deep in the hive, while workers fly about madly and work themselves to death or are snatched up by predators. Those larvae destined to be queens are fed ten times more often than the worker-destined larvae. The nurse bees provide the queens with a diet that is three times higher in fructose and glucose. The volume and sugar content of the diet regulates the secretion of juvenile hormone. "Thus the vastly different life spans of queens versus workers arise from neuroendocrine influences during development that, in turn, derive from nurturing behavior of workers," says gerontologist Caleb Finch.

Among honeybees, the life of a queen is replete with high drama that ends not with death due to old age, but with reginacide. "During their famous nuptial flights," explains Finch, "young queen bees are inseminated by a succession of drones, which explosively pump sperm into the queens' spermatheca and then fall away, leaving part of their endophalus behind. The drones die almost immediately from this gross injury. Queen bees must fertilize all eggs from this store of up to five million sperm, which suffices for many years of fertilizing approximately 200,000 eggs per year. This survival of sperm is as astounding as the longevity and fertility of the queens, and by far exceeds these capacities in domestic fowl and rodents. However, by two to four years the sperm stores are usually depleted, and the queen will then be killed by the workers and replaced. The supersedure, or elimination of senile queens, appears to be triggered by diminished pheromone production or by some other mechanism that enables the constantly attending workers to recognize the insufficiency of fertilized eggs."[13]

Other species use the environment to improve their chances at longevity. Rockfish evade predators in deep, cold water and live 150 years or more. Bristle cone pines elude insects by living at higher altitudes. Some of these trees have been alive more than five thousand years. And some creatures may not age at all.

"Under some circumstances aging may not occur at all," says Finch. "There are a lot of species of fish and other invertebrates that don't seem to have an increased risk of disease or death."

The plant world offers some startling examples of longev-

---

13. Finch, Caleb E., "New Models for New Perspectives in the Biology of Senescence," *Neurobiology of Aging*, Vol. 12, 1991.

ity. A few years ago, Dr. Jane Shen-Miller, a plant physiologist at the University of California at Los Angeles, received seven brown, oval-shaped lotus seeds from the Beijing Institute of Botany. The seeds, about the size of a marble, had been dug from a dry lakebed in China that 1300 years ago had been the site of a lotus lake cultivated by Buddhist monks.

Dr. Shen-Miller filed through the rock-hard shells of four of the seeds. Three of the seeds sent forth tiny green shoots. She then dried and burned the seedlings in order to establish their ages by radiocarbon dating. The oldest was 1,288 years old, another was 694, and the third was 755.

The seeds are the oldest ever known to germinate and have staggering implications for aging research. "This sleeping beauty which was already there when Marco Polo came to China in the thirteenth century must have a powerful genetic system to delay its aging," said Dr. Shen-Miller wonderingly. "It's unbelievable, it could sleep for thousands of years and in four days a little green shoot emerged."

UCLA biochemist Dr. Steven Clarke, an expert on the chemistry of aging, attributed the tiny seed's ability to germinate to its thick shell which protected the seed from air and water, and the presence of a chemical called L-isoaspartyl methyl transferase enzyme, which he first identified in the 1980s. Dr. Clarke believes the chemical, known as a protein repair enzyme, provided the seeds with the ability to "fend off all age-related damage."

Such may be the case when a creature is safe. It continues to repair itself year after year, and it may not age at all. But not all animals are as lucky as the turtle. The lives of most animals in the wild are stressful in the extreme. It's hard enough for many to find a meal, and only marginally easier to avoid becoming one. That sort of everyday life or death stress apparently plays a major role in determining longevity for most living creatures.

Consider the life of an opossum. It is filled with uncertainty. They are not blessed with fearsome claws and teeth. They are neither quick-thinking nor quick-footed. Fair game for automobiles, owls, coyotes, and bobcats, the opossum slinks about in the dark of night, seeking his own meal and hoping to avoid becoming someone else's.

From the moment of birth opossums lead very traumatic lives. Opossums are marsupials, or pouched mammals, and their babies are tiny, about the size of a large ant. Born blind, deaf, hairless, and with only partially developed hind limbs they must hazard a dangerous half-inch journey from the birth opening into the pouch. They do this by clutching and climbing up their mother's belly fur with well-developed front paws. But not every one of the litter makes it. A typical litter may consist of twenty or thirty pups, but mamma has only thirteen nipples in her pouch. Even that number seems optimistic because generally only five to ten babies live to be weaned.

Steven Austad, a professor of zoology at the University of Idaho, has been tracking opossums for many years. His interest was sparked by a mystery that he uncovered when he first started studying the critters.

"When I would capture one," he explains, "it might be in perfect physical health. It looked fit, it looked fat, it looked sassy. Six months later I would catch the same opossum and it looked horrible. It had fallen apart. It would have cataracts, arthritis, lost weight, it limped. It had just fallen apart in an incredible hurry, and I figured I wouldn't be satisfied until I could understand why."

Austad wondered if the hazardous environment was somehow forcing opossums into a pattern of accelerated aging. "Unlike a turtle," he says, "opossums have a dangerous life their entire life. I think of it the same way I think of humans who live under a constant artillery barrage. You have to get your business done in a hurry. That's the only way you get your business done. The way opossums do that is they hurry through everything. They develop in a hurry, they have their kids in a hurry, and one consequence of that is that they age in a hurry."

For Austad, it was a classic example of natural selection having its most powerful effect early in an organism's life. "But as time passes," he explains, "and the organism's passed through more and more danger, then natural selection grows weaker because there are going to be fewer individuals alive for whatever happens late in life to leave any babies. Natural selection can create a very healthy young animal but it has no power over an old animal any more then if we had a gene that killed us at the age of one hundred. It would have no impact on our reproduction, so natural selection couldn't favor the gene or disfavor the gene."

According to Austad, "Life in a hazardous environment therefore means that whether you age or not, you are not going to live very long. That creates favorable conditions for individuals that reproduce in a hurry. Unfortunately one of the side effects of early reproduction seems to be rapid aging."

For Austad, opossums seemed to be a logical subject for study. "Opossums were a good choice because they age very quickly so you didn't have to spend twenty years figuring out whether your experiment worked," he says. "The other thing was that they could carry a large radio collar so that you could follow them throughout their lives, and one of the nicest things is, because they have their young in their pouch, you could mark them right after they were born and follow an individual straight through its life. Now the rationale of my experiment was simply that if we came to a place that had no predators the environment would be much safer for opossums and over enough generations that should have favored the sorts of genes that would slow down aging."

The problem was to find such a natural laboratory where opossums lived their lives at a more leisurely pace, free of the need to constantly look over their shoulders for predators. "If we came to a place that had no predators the environment would be much safer for opossums and over enough generations that should have favored the sorts of genes that would slow down aging."

Austad's search for a sheltered location led him to Sapelo Island, five miles off the Georgia coast. It is one of many barrier islands that dot the coastlines of the Carolinas and Georgia. But most had no opossums. Always a southern delicacy, during the Civil War starving people had hunted them to extinction on every one of Georgia's barrier islands—except Sapelo.

"The fascinating thing about islands," he says, "is that everything changes biologically. And one thing that eventually happens is that the predators disappear. There simply are not big enough prey populations to support them and then once the predators disappear everything changes on the island."

It was the ideal place to see the effect of natural selection on genes. The genetic changes Austad was looking for in aging occur in fewer generations than most people think.

Laboratory experiments in short-lived mammals can generate significant changes in the aging rate in as few as thirty to fifty generations. For an opossum that is only thirty to fifty years. The opossums on Sapelo Island had four thousand years to alter their aging rate because it was that many years ago that Sapelo Island separated from the mainland. Another important criterion was that it is too far from the mainland for opossums to swim there. If they could, then mainland and island opossums would breed together, constantly mixing their gene pools and no specific genetic adaptation to the island environment would take place.

Four-thousand-year-old Sapelo was ideal. A low-lying barrier island, Sapelo is a state-owned wildlife refuge and contains the University of Georgia Marine Institute. The university had done ecological studies and had found small deer, rattlesnakes, and, of course, opossums. Notably lacking were bobcats, pumas, foxes, and all other opossum predators.

Sapelo seemed to fit all of Austad's requirements. The only question was whether they in fact did age more slowly than their mainland relatives. For hundreds of generations, Sapelo Island opossums have evolved independently from their mainland cousins. When Austad first arrived, he discovered the difference in their behavior was literally day and night.

After hundreds of generations with no predators, the Sapelo Island opossums were no longer afraid to come out in the daytime. It was a major behavioral difference from the opossums Austad had studied elsewhere.

Clearly, the island opossums were behaving differently. But were they aging differently? To find out, Austad began to trap opossums around the island. Using radio collars, Austad could learn how quickly island opossums reproduced, how long they lived, and how slowly they aged—all biological patterns determined by natural selection.

The idea of natural selection is simple. If animals differ in any particular behavior or way of doing things, the one that differs in the way that results in the most babies is ultimately going to have the most offspring, and therefore their genes are going to be the ones that survive.

After tracking opossums for two years, Austad made a re-markable discovery. Island opossums live longer than their mainland cousins—in fact, 50 percent longer. They also produce 50 percent fewer young each year. Now the question was why were they living longer? Was it simply the absence of predators? Or was there some deeper biological cause for their longevity? The answer was hidden in their tails.

Austad chose the tendons of the tail as a study tissue, one that was easily accessible and would reveal signs of aging. Tendons are made of collagen, the most common protein in the body.

"The reason that collagen is so interesting is that it is one of those molecules that you have your entire life," explains Austed. "It is never replaced. So like everything that's not replaced it eventually ages. The other reason is that it's everywhere in your body. It's in the tendons and ligaments of humans just like in opossums. But it's also in your skin and all your internal organs. So what happens to collagen is really important in determining what happens to you. It gets stiffer as it gets older and it gets yellowish as well. The aging that goes on in your tendons and ligaments in fact is one of the reasons that there are no eighty-year-old gymnasts.

"So the goal in this opossum research is to use the colla-gen as a sort of marker of physiological aging. It is very easy for me to determine whether the animals on this island live longer than the animals on the mainland. But what I am really interested in is do they physiologically stay younger than on the mainland. And analyzing this collagen in the lab will let me determine that."

To collect the study tissue, Austad makes a small incision in the animal's tail and fishes out a small fiber from the hundreds that comprise a single tendon bundle. He snips it out and drops it into a vial for further study in the laboratory. A drop of superglue closes the wound. If Austad were to capture the same opossum three months later he probably would be unable to find the original incision.

After comparing enough collagen, Austad was astonished to learn that the tissues of island opossums are actually younger. The lack of predators had caused their genes to shift the balance from reproduction to self-repair—transforming every bone, muscle, and fiber to make them age more slowly. "The really fascinating things about these opossums," he concluded, "is that they have changed in a really fundamental way. The genes within each cell of their bodies are operating differently here on the island as a consequence of having lived for generations and generations in this much safer environment."

Indeed, the differences were remarkable. Having lost their fear of predators, the island opossums also lost the need to churn out babies. The reproductive rate of the Sapelo Island opossums typically was four to six pups at a time. Mainland animals usually had litters of six to nine pups. Fewer babies mean less wear and tear on the body. After two years of research Austad was convinced the Sapelo Island opossums were living longer lives. The rate at which collagen aged in the island opossums was also slower than that of the mainland animals.

"There were differences in survival, which you would expect if aging had changed. So reproduction, survival, physiology, everything has slowed down," says Austad. "The island opossums live about 25 percent longer on average. The longest-lived one we have found so far is about 50 percent older than the longest-lived one ever reported on the mainland."

In terms of years, no opossum has ever been found in the mainland population that lived longer than two and a half years. On Sapelo Island Austad has documented opossums that were four years old. And they continue to reproduce. "On the mainland," says Austad, "by their second year of life those few that are still alive are no longer reproducing very efficiently. Whereas for the ones on Sapelo Island there is no difference at all between first year reproduction and second year reproduction."

Like the turtle's shell, Sapelo Island has provided the opossums with the protection that has extended their life spans. "Darwin really discovered that there is a great deal of variation within species, and given enough time and the appropriate environment species can change enormously," notes Austad. "We are not stuck with a single aging rate. Given the appropriate environment and enough time then aging like height, like weight, like skin color, can change to become faster, to become slower, to become anything that the environment dictates."

How has our environment shaped the way we age? Like all species we make trade-offs that are controlled by the genes we inherit from our ancestors. Perhaps the most significant trade-off is in how much of that genetic inheritance is invested in self-repair and how much is invested to produce offspring. The reason is rooted in our evolutionary past.

Five million years ago our species descended from the trees and parted company with other primates. We are still astonishingly close to our relatives—sharing more than 98 percent of our genes with chimpanzees and gorillas. But we live almost twice as long as they do.

But not everyone lives the same length of time. Longevity differs for each individual. A hundred-year-old man may have the arteries of a forty-year-old, and a forty-year-old may collapse and die of a heart attack brought about by the clogged arteries seemingly of a centenarian. Our chronological age is almost never the equivalent of our biological age. Unlike the passage of time, biological aging defies easy measurement.

"What we would like to have," says anatomy professor Leonard Hayflick, "is one or a few measurable biological changes that mirror all other biological age changes without reference to the passage of time, so that we could say, for example, that someone who is chronologically eighty years old is biologically, or functionally, sixty years old." But, because the biological clock that ticks away in each of us does so at a different rate, there is no standard measure for biological age. Nor is there a standard span for all life.

A number of species are governed by genes that spark spectacular flameouts once reproduction has been accomplished. Pacific salmon struggling upstream, their silver bodies flashing in the sunlight as they leap over rocks, ever upwards through rushing waterfalls, running a gauntlet of hazards to return to the place of their birth and spawn, are a classic example of this spectacular death after birth. For once

the females have deposited their eggs and the males fertilized them, the Pacific salmon then die in a matter of weeks in
sudden, cataclysmic fashion, their adrenal glands bulging,
ulcers tearing apart their stomachs, lesions scarring their kid-
neys, their immune systems collapsed.

The effect is to limit each generation to one reproductive
cycle or semelparity. Repeated reproduction, which is the
norm for most species, is called iteroparity. The term comes
from the Greek myth of Semel, one of the foolish human lovers
of Zeus, who demanded he appear to her in all his glory. When
he did she was incinerated by his blazing presence.

Until about twenty-five years ago, semelparity was
thought to be limited to Pacific salmon (Atlantic salmon can
breed many times), certain species of octopi, lampreys, and
annual flowering plants. But in a rain forest near Brisbane,
Australia, a student began to study a tiny marsupial mammal
called the antechinus. With pointed snouts, several pair of
sharp incisors, and rows of cheek teeth, they look very
much like large shrews. Called marsupial mice, the tiny
brown antechinus adult males weigh in at one and three
quarter ounces and the females are even smaller. Babies are
truly tiny, newborns weigh about one-sixteenth of a gram,
the smallest birth weight of a mammal. Unlike other marsupials, the pouch is not enclosed but forms an open cup.
Thus, when a female carries her young, the entire brood is
readily visible on her belly. But what makes the antichenus
truly remarkable is their reproductive cycle. All of the females in a given population give birth within a few days of
each other, usually at the same time each year. After the babies are weaned, the daughters are allowed to stay on in the
nest, but the sons are chased out. They generally move

about a quarter of a mile away and resettle in nests built by unrelated females. Then, during the mating period, the behavior of both males and females becomes stranger than that of any other mammalian species.

The males in the area gather together in areas, dubbed "arenas," in a tree. Females then visit the arenas to mate. "In the final days of the mating period the picture had changed dramatically," wrote Australian zoologists Andrew Cockburn and Anthony K. Lee.[14] "The males were still confining their activity to a few communal nests but were running desperately from one nest to the other, perhaps in search of a nest with a receptive female . . . Seven days later, every male in the entire population was dead."

In their frenzied searches for receptive females, male antechinus stop feeding, lose hair and teeth and one third of their weight during this time. It's not much of a life for either sex. "In all populations we have studied," noted Cockburn and Lee, "males live no longer than eleven and a half months and die at the conclusion of their first rut. Females may live for three years. Most breed only once, but some survive to breed again with the males of their son's generation. Females do not leave the population abruptly but are subject to the gradual attrition that affects most mammals, with death caused by starvation, cold snaps in winter, or predation by owls and nonnative cats and foxes."

Most interesting to biologists, however, is that the cause of death in the males appears to be identical to that of Pacific salmon after they have spawned. Autopsies of male antechi-

---

14. Cockburn, Andrew, and Lee, Anthony K., "Marsupial Femme Fatales," *Natural History,* March 1988.

nus reveal massive gastrointestinal ulcers and a deeply suppressed immune system. "Measurements showed that glucocorticoids (stress hormones) reach extreme levels in males during the mating season," reported Cockburn and Lee.

It's as if nature had waited for the next generation to be assured and then thrown a hormonal death switch. Humans have a similar, although usually less lethal switch triggered by stress. Hormones called hydrocortisones stored in the adrenal glands can trigger a so-called "fight or flight reaction." Under extreme stress, the hormones flood the body, mobilizing glucose, releasing it from storage sites in the body, and pouring it into the blood. At the same time they speed up the heart rate and raise blood pressure to speed the delivery of the glucose to the muscles. Hydrocortisone and glucocorticoids also turn off all kinds of long-term, energy consuming functions that can be shelved until the emergency has passed, such as digestion, growth, reproduction, tissue repair, and the maintenance of the immune system.

"Pacific salmon and marsupial mice meet sudden death when their bodies loose a veritable flood of glucocorticoids," explain Stanford University's Robert Sapolsky and USC's Caleb Finch. "Around the mating period three changes take place that guarantee catastrophe. First, far more glucocorticoids than normal are secreted. Second, the concentration of proteins in circulation that can bind glucocorticoids—in effect sponging them up and buffering organs from the effects of the hormones—falls sharply, allowing the glucocorticoids unrestrained access to target tissues. Finally, part of the brain, as yet unknown, that normally curtails glucocorticoid secretion before too much damage is done fails to function. How all these steps work is poorly understood, but the result is that massive, pathological levels of glucocorticoids pummel the body. The Pacific salmon and the marsupial mice die from the effect of half the stress-related illnesses on earth, packed into a few miserable weeks."

Inexorable as these events appear to be, they can be stopped in their tracks. If the secretion of glucocorticoids is halted just after mating, by removing the adrenal glands, the salmon and the antechinus will live on for a year or more, instead of a stress-plagued few weeks. "The procedure," say Sapolsky and Finch, "demonstrates how drastically the aging process can be affected in otherwise diverse creatures that happen to have evolved the same hormonal death switch."

It also seems to underline the role of natural selection. Since Pacific salmon have fulfilled their genetic imperative and reproduced, their further presence might pitch them into direct competition with their young for food. The antechinus, on the other hand, is born helpless and must have parental care to survive. That care, however, comes from the mother. The male antechinus play no role in child-rearing and, like so many male mammals, are little more than sperm-mobiles racing frantically about in a brief frenzy of mating.

It may at first appear illogical and wasteful of living resources, but it is supremely logical, given the evolutionary imperative to pass on to the next generation the genes that are fittest. And that, in the final analysis, seems to be the ultimate goal of all life.

3 The Genetics of Aging

Thirty million years ago, in what is now the Dominican Republic, a small, stingless bee flew into a tree. Resin weeping out through the bark covered the bee, killing it. The resin containing the bee eventually hardened into amber and was recently cracked open by researchers at the California Polytechnic State University in San Luis Obispo. Inside the stomach of the bee microbiologist Raul Cano found spores of a bacteria he recognized as *Bacillus sphaericus.*

Cano then drew out bacteria from the spores and compared its DNA with that of modern bacteria. There were enough differences to convince him that the bacteria had indeed grown from the ancient spores. The *Bacillus sphaericus* had survived for millions of years without air or nutrients by going into a state of suspended animation. In times of stress, many types of microbes knit themselves a strong, protective shell of protein called a spore and slow all their cellu-

lar processes until they barely maintain life. When temperatures reach life support levels and sufficient nutrients are
available they signal a sort of "bacterial all clear," and the microbes resurrect themselves.

But as Cano found, they don't rouse easily. Even after he
had dissected out the bee's stomach and put its contents in a
petri dish, he still needed to find the precise recipe of metal
ions, amino acids, and other ingredients that would allow the
bugs to awaken and grow. Cano likens the task to reintro-
ducing food to a starving person. "Usually you can't feed him
fettuccine Alfredo," he says. "You have to give him bread and
water and then just sort of work him up to fettuccine."

Cano originally reported that he had revived just one
sleeping species, but he says he's now found more than two
thousand. Among them are several other *Bacillus* species,
several species of the *Actinomyces bacterium*, and even
some 20- to 35-million-year-old yeast.

Many scientists questioned the remarkable age of the bacteria and claimed it was not ancient at all, but rather the product of modern-day contamination of the sample. Dr. Cano
claims to have eliminated the possibility of contamination by
modern bacteria by incorporating several safeguards in the
experiments. The amber surface was first sterilized before it
was cracked open. The entire procedure was conducted
under a decontaminated, Class II laminar flow hood that had
never been used for any other bacterial extraction processes.

The researchers also instituted a number of control measures during the procedure to monitor for external contamination. Pieces of the broken amber were incubated with the
solutions used in the sterilization process for two weeks,
with no evidence of bacteria. Petri dishes containing soy agar

were also placed under the hood throughout the tissue removal process. These control dishes were incubated for two weeks with no evidence of bacterial contamination.

Cano also compared the DNA of the recovered bug with that of modern *B. sphaericus* and concluded they were not close enough to be contemporaries. Similar comparisons were done with other molecular fingerprints. All led him to the same conclusion: the bugs are old.

"It is obvious that micro-organisms are really inveterate survivors," Cano remarks. "They've been surviving and struggling through changing environments for 3.5 billion years. So they must know how to do it."[15]

If Cano's bacteria are indeed thirty million years old they might lead one to the conclusion that immortality, or the next thing to it, is possible, at least on the microbial level. Great age (as opposed to aging) is well known among one-celled organisms. The most likely mechanism responsible is the manner in which one-celled organisms reproduce.

There are essentially two ways living creatures pass their DNA on to the next generation. Large organisms, such as humans and many plants, reproduce by recombining the DNA carried in their germ cells (sperm and egg) into a new organism that inherits a mix of genes from both parents. Bacteria and other single-celled organisms, however, send the next generation on into the world with exactly the same genes as the previous one. Some species such as yeast send out miniature replicas of themselves in the form of buds; others simply split into two equal parts.

Such reproductive behavior is called fission, and some bi-

---

15. *Discover,* January 1996, p. 49.

ologists believe that it confers virtual immortality on those creatures that practice it. How does this apparent immortality fit the evolutionary theory that natural selection favors early reproduction at the cost of subsequent aging of the parents?

"The products of an equal fission are not parent and off-spring," explains Canadian biologist Graham Bell. "They are two new organisms of the same age. Since there are no 'younger' and 'older' individuals, there is no way for increased reproduction by younger individuals to be traded off against survival. The evolutionary theory of aging would predict, therefore, that fissiparous animals do not age."[16]

Bell decided to test the theory by comparing the life cycles of a tiny freshwater worm that reproduces by fission against that of an equally small water flea that reproduces by laying eggs. As Bell expected, the egg-producing fleas aged and died even when maintained in optimal conditions. The freshwater worms also died from time to time, but the rate at which they died did not increase with age. "As the theory predicts," declares Bell, "they seem to be creatures in which senescence is very slow or even entirely lacking."

Studies on similar organisms in the wild are consistent with the results obtained in the laboratory, making reproduction by fission the way to go if something approaching immortality is the ultimate goal. "The longest-lived of all creatures," points out Bell, "are not elephants or tortoises or even large trees but colonies of coral polyps or creosote bushes, which can give rise to new units through a process akin to fission and which may live to an age of thousands or even tens of

---

16. Bell, Graham, "Dividing They Stand," *Natural History,* February 1992.

thousands of years. Here again, where the distinction between parent and offspring breaks down, there is little senescence, just as the evolutionary theory of aging suggests."

Bell's work is one more solid piece of evidence supporting the evolutionary theory of aging. It does not however address the question of whether or not there are specific genes that cause aging. Investigators are finding genetic clues to aging and longevity in very simple organisms such as yeast cells that have some intriguing genetic similarities to human cells. In a laboratory at Louisiana State University, in New Orleans, Michal Jazwinski is studying yeast cells, which can divide only a limited number of times. This allows researchers to observe and calculate the life span of individual cells. Yeast normally have about twenty-one cell divisions or generations. Jazwinski found that over the course of that "life span," certain genes in the yeast are more active or less active as the cells age. They are, in the language of molecular biology, "differentially expressed." So far, Jazwinski has found fourteen such genes in yeast. When one of those genes continued to be active, or, as the geneticists say, "be over-expressed," in some of the yeast cells, the cells went on dividing for twenty-seven or twenty-eight generations; their period of activity was extended by 30 percent.

In his second experiment, Jazwinski mutated the gene, inhibiting its ability to produce a specific protein. When he introduced this non-working version into a group of yeast cells, they had only about twelve divisions. The two experiments made it clear that the gene, now called LAG-1, or Longevity Assurance Gene, influences the number of divisions in yeast or, if you will, its longevity. Just how LAG-1 works is still a mystery. One small clue lies in its sequence of DNA bases—its genetic code—which suggests that it produces a protein found in cell membranes. One next step is to study the function of that protein. Similar sequences have been found in human DNA, so a second investigative path is to clone the human gene and study its function. If there turns out to be a human LAG-1 counterpart, new insights into aging may be uncovered.

At Brown University, in Providence, Rhode Island, a team of researchers led by John Sedivy has uncovered a gene that is a rough equivalent of LAG-1 in human cells. Dubbed p21, this gene disrupted the natural progression of division and death in human cells, endowing the cells with an extended life span.

Using a technique that is routinely used to genetically engineer "knockout" mice for scientific research, the researchers removed the p21 gene from human cells. One of the best ways of studying a gene's role is to remove or knock it out of an organism, thereby eliminating its function. Knockout mice, for example, are used as models of human disease, such as cystic fibrosis, which can be induced in mice by removing one or more of their genes. By removing p21 from ordinary human cells cultivated in the lab the researchers were able to temporarily thwart the aging process. Cells without the gene divide up to thirty additional generations before dying.

"For obvious ethical and medical reasons, we can't make a knockout human, and we're not going to clone a human, so this is as close as we can get," said John Sedivy, an associate professor of molecular biology, cellular biology, and biochemistry at Brown. The adaptation of the knockout method to human cells has broad disease-fighting implications because it allows scientists to study genetically varied human cells without altering human beings to produce such cells.

The Brown research may have important gene therapy implications. "There is no reason we couldn't take cells from a patient, alter them, and put them back in that patient," said Sedivy. "That's exactly what a lot of gene therapy trials are doing now, but they are using less sophisticated methods."

The Brown research also seems to support the ticking clock theory of aging—the idea that a genetic program determines the human life span. "Compelling evidence exists that there is a genetic molecular clock in all cells in the body, irrespective of how you've taken care of yourself," according to Sedivy. "The findings are the best evidence yet that senescence, the mechanism behind growing old, is a real thing. We think we are looking at the molecular mechanism that actually determines senescence. Our goal is to understand and describe that mechanism."

However, the aging process is much more complicated than one gene's activities. "We probably have to alter a bunch of genes before human cells become immortalized," Sedivy said. "But we think this finding is an important incremental step, because there are probably not a lot of genes involved, maybe a half-dozen at most."[17]

While there is no general agreement on just how many genes affect aging in humans, it is also evident that there are several genes that play a role in the aging of yeast. Two, known as RAS1 and RAS2 genes, serve as nutritional sensors keeping the cellular fluids in balance. RAS1 seems to shorten life span, while RAS2 prolongs it. By genetic manipulation in his lab, Jazwinski has over-expressed or continued the activity of RAS2 in yeast, thereby extending its longevity. Another

---

17. *The Brown University News Bureau Report*, September 29, 1997.

gene, PHB1, may play an even greater role and, in fact, be essential for long life. Jazwinski believes there is an additive effect among a number of genes that extend life span, suggesting more than one pathway to longevity.

Jazwinski also found that increasing the yeast's ability to tolerate heat led to a longer life span. However, if heat shock was administered chronically, life span seemed shortened. There is an obvious analogy to human stress.

"Many people believe that chronic stress contributes to human aging," says Jazwinski, "especially brain aging, and only additional research will tell us if chronic stress in yeast will broaden our knowledge of chronic stress in humans."

For the answer to that and other questions of the role genes play in the aging process many biologists have turned to the *Drosophila*, those tiny fruit flies that buzz around bananas. And for good reason—they are small, easily bred, produce a new generation every two weeks, and live for only a month. It is a powerful attraction for a scientist whose own productive life may only be thirty or forty years. Where evolutionary aging theory is concerned, the fruit fly, *Drosophila melanogaster*, as a laboratory tool is well-nigh irresistible.

One of the first people to recognize this was John Maynard Smith, an engineer who spent World War II designing British fighter planes. After the war Smith shifted his remarkable scientific skills to studying the relationship between longevity and reproduction. First he raised several generations of females in isolation from males and found the females laid fewer eggs and lived longer. Next, he sterilized the females and raised them at temperatures high enough to stunt normal egg development. Again, these females lived longer. Finally in an attempt to see whether genetically reduced reproduction would also extend fruit fly life, he selectively bred a group of females who carried a genetic mutation that prevented development of the ovaries. This group lived longest of all.

Smith's experiments lay around the literature for thirty years, interesting but not considered particularly relevant to studies of the aging process in human beings. Then, in 1980, a young evolutionary biologist named Michael Rose, at the University of California at Irvine, fixed upon the idea that aging is genetic and a direct result of evolution. Moreover, he believed he could extend life in fruit flies by delaying the time at which they gave birth. "Aging is not a fixed process. It's nothing fixed, it's nothing absolute from the day you are born. We really understand how it works now. Not all the details, but we really understand it compared to a lot of other biological processes. And from that understanding we know that we can change it."

The goal was ambitious, but the experiment was simple. Fruit flies normally reproduce every fourteen days The females lay their eggs on the food in their cages, but instead of allowing the eggs to hatch, Rose removes the egg-laden food and replaces it. The flies continue to lay eggs that are also removed without hatching. Rose repeats the process— allowing the flies to lay eggs and removing them prior to hatching—for up to ten weeks. Most of the flies die, and those remaining are really old (by fruit fly standards, that is). At this point Rose finally relents and allows the eggs to hatch.

This new generation of flies, born from the oldest of the surviving females, has been selectively bred for longevity. "When you let those flies reproduce," explains Rose, "you are doing two things. The first thing you are doing is you are selecting those flies that live long enough. Because if you wait long enough this cage would be littered with dead flies, some will be alive, some will be dead. The ones that have stayed alive are the ones that obviously are more likely to have the genetic ability to live longer. The second thing you are doing is you are selecting for fertility. Fertility at later ages. So if you only reproduce with these flies at much later ages, a lot of the females are probably infertile and can't reproduce. Those females that can still reproduce at those later ages, those are the females that are going to be the parents of the next generation. In this way from one generation to the next, cumulatively, you produce postponed aging."

The experiment is carried out for a minimum of ten generations. "After ten generations you get an effect," says Rose. "We have taken these old populations here out to over one hundred generations and they are some of the longest-established lines of their kind."

Rose had imposed a new set of rules on nature's game. "Instead of letting them reproduce fast when they are young we delay their reproduction until they are older. By doing that, evolutionary theory tells us we should force evolution to produce an animal that is going to live much longer."

Rose is, in effect, selecting for flies that possess the genes for long life. The tool Rose uses to manipulate the fly's genes is called selective breeding. It's an ancient technique we have used to transform wild animals like the wolf into the many faces of man's best friend. We have used selective breeding to harness the wild horse—enhancing its behavior, power, and speed.

"We select for postponed aging the same way that somebody who owns race horses selects for faster race horses. We make natural selection do the work for us by fiddling with its parameters. By changing the rules under which it operates and then it does all of this work selecting for us and produces an outcome which is the postponed aging animal," says Rose.

After ten years and one hundred generations, Rose has achieved astonishing success. He is the first person to successfully breed long-lived animals. His flies live for as much as ninety-five days. By harnessing the engine of evolution, he has doubled the life span of his flies.

"Natural selection is incredibly powerful," he declares. "It is an unbelievably powerful force. It is the directing, shaping force of all of biology. Once it starts to work on a problem it can make tremendous progress. And that is what we seek in our laboratory—tremendous progress, achieved by natural selection, for which we are happy to take credit."

Having created a long-lived fly, Rose can now investigate how it manages to survive so well. By counting the dead, he can measure how long his flies can live under different kinds of stress.

"It is actually almost science fiction to talk about it, but with our fruit flies we get two- to five-fold improvements in their normal kinds of performances, under very stressful, strenuous conditions. So if you were to think about it in athletic terms it would be like running the hundred meters in half the time or jumping twice as high or four times as high in the high jump."

In effect, Rose has created a race of "superflies" with greater flight endurance. They walk around more when they are older. They store increased caloric reserves in the form of fat for resistance to stress and they are better able to cope with the destructive by-products of their metabolism. When exposed to heat, normal flies die within hours. Rose's flies survive for several days. In dry conditions normal flies die in twelve hours. Rose's live up to five times longer. Normal flies stop mating after fourteen days, while Rose's flies continue mating for up to fifty days.

When scientists first heard of Rose's experiments back in the eighties they presumed the flies increased age mimicked the worst sort of human old age. "One of the common misunderstandings about the kinds of flies that we create in our laboratory is that they are in some way just barely hanging on to life and they are enfeebled and decrepit and just generally crappy, but they somehow manage to survive a long time," recalls Rose. "Sort of the image of everybody's maiden great, great aunt who never did anything with her life and finally died uneventfully. In fact, our flies with postponed aging are completely different from that, and, in fact, one of my favorite examples is to say our flies are like superior athletes, like professional athletes. They can do all kinds of things much better. They can fly much longer when they are tethered and so on."[18]

Rose points with pride to a Plexiglas box. "This is a box in which a whole bunch of flies, thousands of flies are being systematically dried out, many of them to the point of death. Some of them will, in fact, survive this process of severe drying out and the reason why they will survive is because they are resistant to this particular form of stress and more resistant then normal flies. So this is just one physical example of how we make a fly with postponed aging, we make a superior fly. We don't make an inferior fly that drags it all out

---

18. In the laboratory flies are tethered, or tied by a strong thread to a post, and the number of times their wings beat and other attributes of flying ability can be measured.

longer, instead we make a superior fly, which is robust enough to go on living, and in fact it is more robust than normal for much of its life, and it's only toward the end of its life that it starts to undergo a process of pervasive deterioration the way almost all animals do. So this is our one example of our basic conviction that to postpone aging means to enhance health and enhance performance and enhance your basic capacity to live.

"At ages where almost all the normal flies are dead, the majority of our flies with postponed aging are busy reproducing, walking around, and having a great time. So it is a very radical transformation," says Rose.

By preventing early reproduction, Rose has transformed the flies' genes—extending self-repair for far longer than normal. To Rose, these flies prove that human aging can be altered in ways that surpass current aging remedies. And the possibilities for human longevity are staggering.

"Running more, eating less, eating more fruit, eating more vegetables, eating more nuts, eating less nuts, whatever, all of those things might buy you a year or two here and there. It might keep your prostate ticking over a little while longer. Delay the onset of cancer by nine months to eighteen months and so on. Maybe. We don't even know that that's true but let's concede that. What we are talking about with our research, with applying the evolutionary theory of aging, with what we have accomplished with our organisms in the laboratory is doubling life span, potentially tripling life span. We our talking about the difference between dynamite and atomic weapons," states Rose emphatically.

Imagine record-breaking athletes who are fifty or sixty years old but look like they are twenty-five. Imagine everyone you know is twice their age but look no older than they are today. Imagine having babies at 70, being fit and healthy until the very end of life at 150, or perhaps 200.

Such profound biological change is now a possibility. To make it a reality, scientists are searching for genes that control human aging. That search is but a part of one of the most important explorations ever attempted by humankind. It is in its boldness and goals as visionary as Columbus's search for a passage to India, as the Apollo project. Called the Human Genome Project, its goal is no less than the complete mapping and understanding of all the genes that make up the human body. Sequencing the eighty to one hundred thousand genes that comprise the human genome should be completed by 2005.

Consider that forty years ago, the structure of DNA had just been solved and the precise number of human chromosomes was still under debate. The major research tool was a state-of-the-art computer that weighed in at thirty tons and covered about one thousand square feet of floor space. Since then we have learned that there are forty-six human chromosomes, which between them house three billion base pairs of DNA and encode about sixty to eighty thousand proteins. These coding regions make up only about 2 percent of the genome (the function of the remaining 98 percent is unknown), and some chromosomes have a higher density of genes than others. One of the most difficult challenges ahead is to find genes involved in diseases that have a complex pattern of inheritance, such as those that contribute to diabetes, cancer, heart disease, and the aging process. Researchers have already identified single genes associated with a number of diseases, such as Alzheimer's disease, cystic fibrosis,

Duchenne muscular dystrophy, myotonic dystrophy, neu-rofibromatosis, and retinoblastoma.

With more complete understanding of the human genome will come the ability to prevent or repair genetic damage at the cellular level, thought to be a major cause of aging. Nor will the application of this new genetic understanding stop there. A virtual explosion of gene therapy applications to medical problems will very likely bring hitherto intractable diseases under control. As research progresses, investigators will also uncover the mechanisms for diseases caused by several genes or by a single gene interacting with environmental factors. The identification of these genes and their proteins will pave the way to more effective therapies and preventive measures. Investigators determining the underlying biology of genome organization and gene regulation will also begin to understand how humans develop from single cells to adults, why this process sometimes breaks down, and what changes take place as people age.

Biologists who study evolution have long thought that many genes suddenly gone awry at the same time are responsible for the aging process. Aging is controlled by a multitude of genes, says their theory, and it is therefore impossible to think of the process as a simple disease to be cured by some single genetic manipulation or intervention.

But that theory is under attack by molecular biologists who work at the genetic and cellular level. "The identification of genes that slow the rate of aging has made people recognize that the fundamental aging process, even in higher organisms, could be under genetic control and can maybe be modulated," says Dr. Thomas E. Johnson, a biologist at the University of Colorado.

In the fruit fly, one such gene has been found. The next question is what genes and what gene products are involved? Since the first experiments, Rose has bred longer life spans into fruit flies by selecting for other characteristics, such as ability to resist starvation, so the flies' long life spans are not necessarily tied to their fertility late in life.

In another laboratory at the University of California at Irvine, the late Robert Tyler and James Fleming, a molecular biologist, discovered that the longer-lived flies had a somewhat different form of a gene that orders production of the enzyme superoxide dismutase. The SOD gene was more active than its counterpart in the flies with average life spans. SOD scavenges the body for oxygen radicals that tear up normal cells. The enzyme links to the oxygen and starts a process that eventually converts the molecules to water. Simply by inserting a gene that codes for an extremely active form of the enzyme, Fleming extended the life span of normal flies by 10 percent. This finding has given a boost to the hypothesis that antioxidant enzymes like SOD are linked to aging and longevity. (See Chapter Four.)

Some of the genes found in yeast and fruit flies seem to promote longevity. But others may shorten life span. One such "death gene" has been isolated in *Caenorhabditis elegans*. The animal is among the most intensely studied organisms in nature, a transparent, microscopic roundworm known as a nematode. It is one of the geneticist's favorite laboratory tools. Barely a millimeter long, about the size of the comma in this sentence, it is also common as dirt. A shovelful from your backyard will contain millions of nematodes.

Researchers at the Institute of Behavioral Genetics at the University of Colorado in Boulder found that mutation of a certain gene more than doubles the nematode's normal three-week life span. Thomas Johnson's laboratory in Boulder has also uncovered evidence that the mutant may extend life span by overproducing SOD and catalase, two antioxidant enzymes that have been linked to longevity in other studies.

The genes isolated so far are only a few of what scientists think may be dozens, perhaps hundreds, of longevity and aging-related genes. Tracking them down in organisms like nematodes and yeast is just the beginning. The next big question for many gerontologists is whether there are counterparts in people—human homologues—of the genes found in laboratory animals.

The genetic leap from simple organisms such as yeast and worms to humans is at first glance gargantuan and seemingly beyond all meaningful extrapolation. But recent work at Stanford University has plotted the entire genomes of two yeast and nematode worms along the same evolutionary pathway that leads to plants and animals. The comparison has given genetics researchers still more evidence that the genes of laboratory organisms such as yeast, worms, and fruit flies can be used to reliably predict the function of newly discovered human genes.

"This study represents an important advance," said David Botstein, Ph.D., a professor of genetics at Stanford University School of Medicine and senior author of the study. "It shows that we can learn the function of worm genes from the yeast, and vice versa, which makes it likely that we can also learn the function of conserved human genes from either of these organisms."[19]

---

19. *Science,* December 11, 1998.

The findings show that most of the core biological functions in the unicellular yeast, commonly known as baker's yeast, and the multicellular nematode worm are performed by proteins similar in sequence and number, indicating that protein functions identified in one species can be assigned to the other. Linking similar gene sequences and protein functions in organisms as disparate as yeast and worms paves the way for similar comparisons in all organisms—from yeast to worms, fruit flies, mice, and humans, the researchers said.

The scientists compared the 6,217 yeast genes with the 19,099 genes of the nematode worm. They found that 40 percent of the yeast and 20 percent of the worm sequences code for highly conserved proteins that carry out biological processes common to both microorganisms—such as DNA and RNA metabolism and protein folding, trafficking, and degradation. These proteins show one-to-one relationships, suggesting that the genes encoding them were present and their functions were already established in the common ancestor of fungi and animals.

Specialized processes unique to the worm use novel proteins characteristic of multicellular plants and animals. It is largely these specialized genes that make the worm genome three times the size of the yeast.

At almost the same time as the genetic pathways of the two primitive organisms were being compared, two teams of biologists headed by John E. Sulston of the Sanger Center, near Cambridge, England, and Robert H. Waterston of Washington University, in St. Louis, successfully deciphered the entire gene sequence of the nematode. It has taken ten years to decode the complete nematode genome. When finally unraveled the researchers found its full DNA composed of ninety-seven million chemical units packed into an estimated 19,099 genes. If printed in ordinary type, the DNA sequence would take up 2,748 pages of a daily newspaper. By contrast, the human DNA contains upwards of three billion molecular pairs locked into eighty thousand proteins. To date, only about 7 percent of the human genome have been mapped.

The worm genome has given biologists their first sight of the information needed to develop, operate, and maintain a multicellular animal. Until now, the only genomes that had been sequenced have been those of single-celled organisms like bacteria and yeast.

Since we have learned that worms and humans share many genes in common, the worm genome is regarded by biologists as an essential basis for understanding how the human genome works. "In the last ten years we have come to realize humans are more like worms than we ever imagined," said Dr. Bruce Alberts, president of the National Academy of Sciences. "Seeing the worm's complete genome is humbling, because it makes biologists realize how much there is yet to understand. We always underestimate the complexity of life, even of the simplest processes. So this is really only the beginning of unraveling the mystery of life."

Dr. Eric Lander, director of a human genome sequencing center at the Whitehead Institute at MIT in Cambridge, Massachusetts, said of the findings: "This is really a landmark achievement. It is the first time we've had a picture of the gene set needed to run a multicellular organism.... This is a brilliant innovation of half a billion years ago that we are getting a look at for the first time," referring to the evolution of animals from their single-celled precursors.[20]

Learning the arrangement of the chemicals that make up the DNA molecule, a process known as sequencing, is a time-consuming task. A major problem is that the machines that analyze DNA can read segments of only five hundred units or so in length. The full genome must be fitted together from an inordinate number of small overlapping pieces. Another problem is that the DNA must be copied, or, as the biologists say, amplified, many times to give the machines a sufficient amount to analyze it.

For biologists using the nematode to study the aging process, virtually all of the genetic blanks are now filled in. But even before the last sugar and phosphate of the nematode DNA chains were identified, geneticists like Tom Johnson at the University of Colorado were on remarkably intimate terms with the tiny worms.

"Nematodes," he explains, "are a very simple animal. They have just under a thousand cells. We know the names of each one of those cells; what their functions are, so on and so forth. The distribution of cell types in the worm is remarkably similar although more limited to what one would see in a mammal. They have nerve cells, they have muscle cells. There are remarkable similarities. They have a gut running the length of the animal. Food is ingested through a mouth and excreted through an anus at the other end, just as in

---

20. Wade, Nicholas, "Animal's Genetic Program Decoded, in a Science First," *The New York Times,* December 11, 1998.

higher organisms. This isn't meant to say that the animals are identical, they are by no means identical, and there are a number of cell types that aren't found. There isn't a concrete heart, for instance. These animals are so small that they don't need a heart to circulate blood through them but there are remarkable similarities, and when one gets to the subcellular level, or cellular level, the similarities become even more obvious. The cells are nucleated just as mammalian cells. There are very similar proteins found in the nucleus. The chromosome structure is very similar. So there is remarkable convergence at the cellular and molecular level due to the fact that all life on Earth is evolutionarily related."

Johnson is using those similarities to unravel some of the genetic secrets of human aging. "The little animals that we work on have life spans of only two weeks, and their reproduction period under those conditions is only about eight days," he says. "So they go on and they live another week longer than they need to as far as evolution is concerned. We think that the reason that they go on and continue living is just because they are so well-adapted for this very short life span that they have, that the rest of their life is sort of gravy. So what we are interested, really, in understanding, is why they live longer than that one-week period."

Johnson began by eliminating genes to see if that would actually lead to the animals living longer than normal. Eventually, he found that by eliminating a single gene, which he dubbed "Age 1," the nematodes lived longer. That led to the surprising conclusion that the eliminated genes were actually deleterious. Their normal function was to shorten the life span of the nematode.

"What we are doing now is trying to understand the nature

of that deleterious effect," says Johnson. "What it looks like in our early observations is that these genes are actually making the animals less long-lived by reducing their ability to withstand environmental stresses." When Johnson eliminated the gene, the worm lived about 70 percent longer, and it became more resistant to various stresses.

Johnson's conclusion that "a single gene mutation could lead to increased longevity," initially produced a goodly bit of skepticism in the scientific community. "One of the reasons that people were fairly skeptical of this observation," he recalls, "was the quite valid expectation by evolutionary biologists that hundreds of genes should be involved. For instance, Michael Rose has shown that his fruit flies that live two-fold longer than normal are the result of changes in literally hundreds of different genes. And we expected that that would be in the nematode as well."

But the fact that a single gene was capable of having so great an effect called for a new look at the control mechanism of genetic expression. Johnson concluded that his single gene was a "master gene" capable of coordinating and controlling hundreds of different genes that were in effect downstream from the mutated gene.

"If we think of it as a hierarchy," he explains, "the genes that we have identified as single genes are the generals, and the instructions from the generals are mediated by a hierarchy through colonels, lieutenants, and so forth down to the foot soldier that is actually doing the work, that is creating the environment that is more resistant to these environmental stresses.

"So initially when we were seeking genes that actually led to a longer than normal life span, I was hoping to get handles, molecular handles on the aging process. By doing that now, by lengthening life span we think that we have actually altered the rate of aging, if you will, and that these animals are in a sense aging slower. So the next question then is what drives that slower aging rate? How have we slowed the rate of aging of these animals? And we think that we have done that by increasing the ability of these animals to withstand normal everyday environmental stresses."

Johnson's goal is to discover a gene that affects humans in a similar way. These genes have not yet been found, but many scientists have joined the quest to find them. At McGill University in Montreal, Siegfried Hekimi and Bernard Lakowski have found four genes that when mutated seem to act as biological clocks that slow down every aspect of the nematode worm's life cycle. Called clk-1, mutations in this gene caused individual cells to divide more slowly and as a consequence to develop more slowly. Indeed, every aspect of the life cycle was slowed. The rhythms of nematode life moved at a much more stately pace, the worms ate less and defecated less, even wiggling their bodies less as they swam. And, like Tom Johnson's nematodes, they too lived much longer.

They metabolized food the same way their normal counterparts did, but they used the energy from that food more efficiently, probably spending less energy per unit time. "It shows there is such a thing as a central biological clock which puts into synchrony everything that has a temporal component," says Hekimi.[21]

---

21. Pennisi, Elizabeth, "Worm Genes Imply a Master Clock," *Science,* May 17, 1996, p. 948.

Since their original discovery in 1996, Hekimi and Lakowski have found two more apparent clock genes, dubbed clk-2 and clk-3. Nematodes with combinations of all the clock genes lived three to four times longer than normal. Yet another group of genes found in nematodes can also extend the worm's life. Called daf genes, they regulate the path the maturing larvae take on its way to adulthood. Activated by food shortages or overcrowding, some of the daf genes will sidetrack development into a dormant state known as a dauer stage. When activated, the daf genes can also prolong the life of an adult nematode.

When Hekimi and Lakowski combined a clock gene mutation with a daf gene mutation, the worms lived an astonishing five times longer than normal—the greatest increase in mean life span ever seen in any organism. A similar life extension in a human being would be the equivalent of 420 years. Living to the beat of a slower drummer would appear then to lengthen life.

"These genes seem to set the rate of metabolism and the rate at which things happen. Every kind of periodic or temporal process is slowed down," says Cynthia Kenyon, a geneticist and developmental biologist at the University of California, San Francisco.[22] One of the best-known researchers in the field, Kenyon was one of the ten scientists involved in the March 1999 conference in Los Angeles who attempted to gauge the progress of aging research to that point.

Hekimi sees in the clock genes a single explanation for a rate of living, but many aging researchers don't agree. "There is no one mechanism of aging," says Huber Warner

---

22. Pennisi, Elizabeth. "Worm Genes Imply A Master Clock."

of the National Institute of Aging. "There's both genetic and environmental factors."

Among those environmental factors that affect all living things is the food supply. Some species alter their rate of reproduction based upon the food supply, others raise or lower their rate of metabolism when food is more or less plentiful. In the nematode, nature has provided a gene that governs its life span. When food is plentiful, the worm lives fast and dies young. In lean times, *C. elegans* slams on the metabolic brakes, going into virtual hibernation to conserve energy.

The gene that governs this activity, daf-2, regulates glucose (sugar) metabolism in the nematode. It was discovered by Dr. Gary Ruvkun, a researcher at the Massachusetts General Hospital and Harvard University in Boston. He, like Hekimi and Lakowski in Montreal, speculates that a downshifting of glucose metabolism in times of stress helps the worm live longer.

Dr. David Finkelstein, of the National Institute of Aging's Biology of Aging Program, says, "This finding suggests that altering glucose metabolism could be a key to slowing aging in higher organisms, even perhaps in humans." The daf-2 gene is in the same family of proteins as the receptor that binds insulin in humans; it functions as a switchboard for signals coming into the cell which tell the cell how much food is available. If not enough food or insulin is available, the daf-2 gene swings open a pathway that puts the organism into a hibernating state. A similar decrease in metabolism has been observed in calorically restricted rats. These reduced diets are known to extend life span not only in rats but also in other animals, as we will see in Chapter Four. The inescapable implication is that this same mechanism in humans may provide a means for slowing down aging.[23]

Virtually all researchers agree that there are likely to be hundreds of genes involved in human aging—one of which was discovered at about the same time as the McGill work was being announced. The gene is responsible for Werner's syndrome, a disease that speeds up the aging process in children, producing the exact opposite effect of the nematode clock genes.

Werner's syndrome is a rare genetic disorder that locks its young victims in the bodies of the very old. There are actually two versions of the condition. One, called progeria, afflicts children until about the age of thirteen. Some sixty children have been located with progeria. All were small, bald, wizened, and tragically aware of the savagery of their disease. A rapidly advancing arteriosclerosis usually kills them by the age of thirteen. An adult form of Werner's syndrome begins after puberty. It is a rare disorder that affects about ten of every million people throughout the world. Its victims begin to age dramatically. By the time they are twenty they have developed many of the ills of old age— gray hair, cataracts, wrinkled skin, osteoporosis, and a host of other age-related diseases. By the time they are in their forties most die of heart attacks or cancer.

The syndrome is named for Otto Werner, a German physician who in 1904 published a report about a family affected by premature aging. Werner suggested that the problem was somehow genetic. In 1996, the gene that causes Werner's

---

23. "Altered Genes, Altered Metabolism—Longer Life?" NIA Report, August 1997.

syndrome was found on the short arm of chromosome 8 of the twenty-three pairs of human chromosomes. It was discovered by a team of scientists led by Dr. George Schellenberg of the Veterans Affairs Puget Sound Health Care System and Dr. George Martin, a pathologist at the University of Washington in Seattle.

The Werner's gene is responsible for an enzyme that is essential to DNA function. Called helicase, the enzyme straightens out the twisted strands of DNA. This untwisting is the crucial first step for all DNA functions, such as cell repair, copying itself, and translating DNA code into the proteins that create new cells. When the gene is faulty, the results are a rapid acceleration of the aging process.

The effects of the Werner's gene can be seen on the cellular level. "In a young child," notes Schellenberg, "the cells will divide up to sixty or seventy times. If you take cells from an older person, they only copy ten or twenty times. Their cells stop dividing. A thirty-year-old Werner's patient's cells look like an eighty-year-old. It's become the model of human aging."

To get Werner's, you need two bad copies of the gene. Parents and sibling with only one mutant copy of the gene seem perfectly normal. "The discovery that the mutation involves a member of the helicase family of genes points to the importance of DNA metabolism as a mechanism for the generation of such diverse pathologies as cataracts, osteoporosis, cancer, and forms of arteriosclerosis," says Martin.

Both Schellenberg and Martin were quick to point out that they did not believe it was the only gene responsible for human aging. "I don't think this gene is the aging gene," says Schellenberg. "Aging is more complicated than that." "No single gene could possibly cause aging or all the disorders associated with aging," adds Martin. Nonetheless, the discovery of the gene was considered a major step forward.

"It's the only real model of human aging that we have," said Anna McCormick, chief of the Biology Branch of the National Institute of Aging. "It may not give us all the answers to aging, but we hope it gives us some."[24]

Answers are also coming from other unexpected sources. Consider Helen Boley, a sixty-one-year-old retired Missouri state employee who carries what some researchers are calling a "Methuselah gene." Every Tuesday a vial of Boley's blood is drawn and rushed to the National Heart Lung and Blood Institute in Bethesda, Maryland. Every six months, Boley presents herself in person to the Bethesda Institute.

The reason for all this interest is her HDL, the so-called good cholesterol. In Boley's blood, the HDL levels are off the chart. Dr. William Harris, director of the lipid laboratory at the University of Kansas Medical Center, discovered that Boley has the highest level of HDL ever recorded. Her HDL is 230, more than four and a half times higher than normal.

The remarkable HDL level and the fact that she has unusually long-lived relatives going back three generations has made the sprightly eighty-nine-pound woman an on-going source of medical wonder and study, so much so that Brian Brewer, chief of the Institute's molecular disease branch, has assigned seven researchers to Boley's blood. "She's really unique. We've been looking for someone like her for years," he says. "In a sense, she has an anti-aging gene."

In fact she probably has inherited a double helping of the

---

24. United Press International, April 11, 1996.

same gene that regulates HDL production. If the scientists can unlock the secret of how the gene works, it would lead to totally new ways to protect people from atherosclerosis and the other cholesterol-mediated conditions that lead to heart disease.

Cholesterol is a soft, odorless, waxy substance. The body needs cholesterol to function normally. It is, for example, a component of cell membranes and essential for the production of many hormones, vitamin D, and bile acids, which are important for the absorption of fat. Cholesterol is present in all parts of the body, including the brain and nervous system, muscle, skin, liver and intestines, heart, skeleton, and other parts.

Blood cholesterol level is affected not only by the saturated fat and cholesterol in the diet, but also by the cholesterol the body produces naturally. The problem is since the body produces all the cholesterol it needs, the saturated fat and cholesterol in the diet only serve to increase blood cholesterol levels.

Cholesterol travels in blood packages called lipoproteins. All lipoproteins are formed in the liver and carry cholesterol through out the body. Blood cholesterol packaged in low density lipoproteins (LDLs) is transported from the liver to other parts of the body where it can be used. LDLs carry most of the cholesterol in the blood, and if not removed from the blood, cholesterol and fat can build up in the arteries contributing to atherosclerosis. This is the reason LDL cholesterol is often called "bad cholesterol."

Cholesterol is also packaged in high density lipoproteins. HDLs carry cholesterol back to the liver for processing or removal from the body. HDLs, therefore, help remove cholesterol from the blood, preventing the accumulation of cholesterol in the walls of the arteries. Thus, they are often called "good cholesterol."

A high LDL cholesterol level or a low HDL cholesterol level increases the risk of coronary heart disease. Coronary heart disease is the leading cause of death and disability for both men and women. More than 50 percent of all adults in America have an increased risk of coronary heart disease because of elevated cholesterol levels. An astonishing 57 percent of adult Americans have borderline high or high total cholesterol concentrations and are prime candidates for heart attacks and strokes.

Part of the problem is the average American diet is about 35 to 40 percent fat, of which 15 to 20 percent is saturated. But experts warn that less than 10 percent of calories should come from saturated fat. Individuals of course differ in the speed with which body metabolism removes cholesterol from the bloodstream and how much new cholesterol is manufactured by the liver. But one thing that affects everyone equally is the fact that as they grow older, total blood cholesterol levels will naturally tend to rise.

And that is what makes Helen Boley's HDL levels so fascinating to researchers. For HDL, they have learned, has the ability to check the damage to cells caused when free radicals are produced by the body's burning of oxygen to power those self-same cells. (See Chapter Four.) Some of the damage occurs in the cells that line the arterial walls, leading to the dangerous deposit of fatty plaques. When the plaque deposits build up enough to block or even reduce the flow of blood through the artery, heart attacks or strokes may result.

Boley's genetic gift that enables her to produce HDL in

such astounding quantities also gives her a remarkable ability to shield her cells from the ravages of free-radical oxidation. "She's preventing oxidation damage like crazy," says Dr. Harris. "Her arteries probably are squeaky clean."

For most people, the likelihood of inheriting a genetic program that will insure longevity is minimal. Diet is certainly one way to increase the odds and reduce the risk of many life-shortening diseases such as heart disease, stroke, and cancer. Diet is, in fact, for some gerontologists, one of the main pathways to extending life.

4   *Extending Life*

"**T**he science of aging, that is of life extension, is really the oldest science," says seventy-four-year-old Dr. Roy Walford, a professor of pathology at the University of California at Los Angeles Medical School. "It was invented by the Taoists five thousand years ago, and to extend life span they invented pharmacology, for example. It has gotten exciting recently because finally after thousands of years we are within range of being able to regulate the rate of aging."

Walford is a true believer in extending life by diet—specifically and very simply by reducing the amount of food we eat, by restricting calories. Caloric Restriction or the CR-diet was first developed in 1935 by Clive M. McCay, a researcher at Cornell University. Low in calories but high in nutrients, the diet has a surprising and dramatic effect on health. McCay found he could extend the lives of laboratory rats by about 50 percent simply by cutting their calories to near-starvation levels.

The significance of these findings was virtually ignored until the early 1970s when Walford not only began to reproduce McCay's experiments but undertook to learn why near-starvation could achieve such dramatic results in longevity.

In his lab at UCLA he has, over the course of the last twenty-five years, put thousands of mice to the test. In each experiment, half of the mice, the control group, eat all they want. The other half receive 40 percent fewer calories—but all the nutrients they need. The results have been quite remarkable and, Walford believes, offer a significant and yet simple means of extending human life.

"What these mice have given mankind is perhaps the answer to a healthier, longer life," he says. "They live a remarkable one-third longer than their well-fed counterparts. This is the first and only intervention proven to extend maximum life span throughout the animal kingdom."

In fact, in every species in which caloric restriction has been tested, longer life has been the end result. "It works all the way across the animal kingdom," declares Walford. "Calorically restricted one-celled organisms, worms, mice, rodents, rats, fish, all live a great deal longer, equivalent to, let's say, 150 to 160 years in humans. So it would be very surprising if it worked all across the animal kingdom and then not in humans.

"The second piece of evidence is, as I showed in the Biosphere 2 experiment, humans when they are calorically restricted showed the same extensive physiologic, biochemical, hormonal, and blood changes that rodents do when they are calorically restricted. What these two pieces of evidence together show is that it's almost certain that it will work in humans."

In a well-publicized experiment in 1991, Walford, three other men, and four women were sealed inside Biosphere 2 in the desert outside of Tucson, Arizona. The domed structure covered three acres and served as an encapsulated replica of the Earth's ecosystems, containing everything from marshlands and desert, ocean and farmland. Like so many discoveries in science, what happened next was the work not of planning but of serendipity. The cleverly constructed, carefully planned Biosphere failed to yield enough food for the intrepid "guinea pigs" to eat a normal diet.

"It was kind of miraculous that someone of my background happened to be the medical officer," says Walford. "An ordinary nutritionist would have freaked out and insisted that food be brought in."

Walford, however, saw it as an opportunity to replicate his mice experiments with human subjects who, like their rodent counterparts, were in no condition to argue. For the next six months Biosphereans, ranging in age from twenty-eight to Walford's then sixty-seven, lived on a diet of only 1800 calories. The average American consumes between 2500 and 3500 calories a day. The minimal diet and the hard physical labor needed to keep their domed world running left them hungry, but increasingly lean and fit. The men showed an average weight loss of twenty-six pounds, the women fifteen pounds. By every measure they were healthier. Blood pressure fell sharply. Total cholesterol dropped a remarkable 35 percent on average, even for those who began with low levels. The drop, in fact, exceeded anything previously achieved by either diet or drugs, according to Walford. And, as had been noted in calorically restricted animal experiments, there was a large drop in white blood cell counts indicating a strong immune system.

Another significant finding was the Biosphere 2 people exhibited some of the same changes found in hibernating animals. Their body temperatures were slightly lowered and other physiologic changes were noted. But not all of the hibernating similarities were attributed to caloric restriction. "Besides the food restriction," notes Walford, "we also were deprived, to a considerable extent, of oxygen during the experiment. The oxygen in Biosphere 2, for various reasons declined gradually, so we were low in oxygen, low in food intake. The changes in our blood, compared to what oxygen deprived humans show in high altitudes, were opposite to what was expected in our blood hemoglobin and certain enzyme values. However, in hibernating animals, say, turtles that bury under the mud in rivers and hibernate, it was more like that. Their blood changes in terms of these hemoglobin values were the same as ours. Hibernating animals are food-deprived and oxygen-deprived. And we were, too, we showed the same changes.

"The significance of the experiment," concluded Walford, "was that humans get the same physiological response as animals do." And that he believes also means that humans will live longer on a calorically restricted diet.

In fact, he has no such doubts where his own life is concerned, thriving on a nutrient-rich 1700 calories a day—30 percent less than normal for a man of his size and age.

"I've been calorie-restricted for eight or ten years. I expect if I keep this up that it will add fifteen to twenty years to my life span. I think that diet is very healthy and it makes you feel better. I need less sleep. You have more energy, but you are little hungry. But I'm a lot hungrier to live longer for knowledge, beauty, and justice, and things like that than I am for angel food cake. So it's a good substitution."

The calorie-restricted diet has certainly done wonders for his mice. Walford's mice live about 44 percent longer than the control group and even longer when compared to mice in the wild.

To test the strength of these long-living mice, Walford invented a log-rolling contest. He discovered, somewhat surprisingly, that these calorie-restricted mice also had more stamina and were more nimble than their well-fed counterparts. Placing a restricted mouse and a more portly, control group mouse on a wooden rod extending above the cage floor, the mice scramble to stay on top of the "log."

"This restricted one," Walford points out, "does better on the log-rolling test, he has better coordination and muscular control than the fully fed mouse. So he is younger in physiology than the other one, although they are both the same chronological age. One can also see if you compare the two mice that the calorically restricted mouse is more active, he is about to bite me if he can, and his coat is more shiny than the controlled mouse."

In fact Walford's restricted mice seem altogether healthier. They have better immune systems and fewer age-related diseases. Despite all the evidence pointing to the benefits of caloric restriction, however, the specific mechanism by which it works its presumed wonders is not completely understood. The problem, Walford points out, is that it fits all of the theories of aging quite well.

"It increases DNA repair, it prevents the formation of so many free radicals and perhaps up-regulates the body's own antioxidant systems. It prevents the age-related decline in the immune system. It lowers blood sugar·and...corresponds with some of the hormonal changes. And so it has an embarrassment of possibilities. It fits every theory of aging. It even fits the evolutionary theory quite well, because we think that it's basically an adaptive response whereby animals, when faced with periodic food shortages, change their energy from growth and reproduction into maintenance and repair and so survive the periods of food shortage."

Will caloric restriction lead to longer life for humans? It's too early to tell—but the goal is as much for quality as it is for quantity. For lurking in the dim background of longevity research is the frightening echo of ancient myth. In the Greek legend, Eos, the goddess of dawn, asked Zeus to bestow eternal life on her mortal lover Tithonus. Zeus did as bid, but Eos had not fully thought out the consequences of her request. Tithonus lived on and on, but he fell apart along the way, becoming withered and wizened, senile and decrepit—ultimately shriveling into a grasshopper. It was the ultimate and perhaps the first catch-22: Eos had neglected to ask for eternal youth for Tithonus to accompany her request for eternal life.

"The goal," explains Walford, "is to create people that may be a hundred in chronological years, but that test out and look and feel in every way like a person of present-day forty years of age. So we're not extending merely a bunch of frail, old years, but the period of youth and vitality, middle age, and the young-old period. So the last ten years of life today from eighty to ninety, let's say, will in future be 140 to 150."

Walford acknowledges that in the future there will be simpler methods to extend life span and retard aging than caloric restriction. "These will involve genetic manipulation," says Walford. "There are genes known in certain animals, and if you regulate those or control them you can extend life span. That's one approach. There are also probably things that one can take in the future in the form of a pill that will prevent free radical damage and other ways to prevent damage from glycation. So I think the future will present easier methods than calorie restriction. But if you want to hang around for the future, calorie restriction is the only thing known to work now."

There are only about 150 or 200 people around the world who are known to actually be on a calorically restricted diet similar to Dr. Walford's. That is too small a group and they have not lived long enough on the diet to say unequivocally that CR (calorie restriction) is unquestionably the key to 120-year life spans. But there are some intriguing findings that have been made among small isolated population groups around the world.

"Consider the people of Okinawa, many of whom consume diets that are low in calories but provide needed nutrients," says Dr. Rick Weindruch, a former graduate student of Walford's, now at the University of Wisconsin. "The incidence of centenarians there is high—up to forty times greater than that of any other Japanese island. In addition, epidemiological surveys in the United States and elsewhere indicate that certain cancers, notably those of the breast, colon, and stomach, occur less frequently in people reporting small caloric intakes."[25]

Moreover, studies of monkeys—among our closest ge-

---

25. Weindruch, Richard, "Caloric Restriction and Aging," *Scientific American,* January 1996.

netic cousins—are proving to be similar to those achieved by Dr. Walford in his mouse experiments. One of the major research projects in the field is led by Dr. Weindruch at the University of Wisconsin Regional Primate Research Center in Madison. He is conducting new work in caloric restriction—getting one step closer to applying the science to humans. Weindruch heads the largest, long-term caloric restriction study of its kind on rhesus monkeys.

"We don't know for sure if it corresponds to humans," says Weindruch. "That's one reason we're doing studies in monkeys—to see if the kinds of things we observe in the mice and rats actually happen in a species that's very closely related to us."

A favorite for aging studies, the rhesus monkey also happens to be the most commonly studied non-human primate in all of biology. At the Wisconsin Regional Primate Center the rhesus monkey colony was established more than forty years ago, providing researchers with what Weindruch believes is "one of the world's largest colonies of 'old' rhesus monkeys."

The study, which began in 1989, consists of seventy-five monkeys divided into a calorie-restricted group and a control group given license to eat everything that is offered to them. Since rhesus monkeys will live for thirty to forty years, the experiment is still in its early stages.

"Our oldest animals now are only twenty years of age and have been on the diet for about eight years maximum," explains Weindruch. "We still have to wait another fifteen or so years to know about the longevity effects, because this is a species which can live as long as forty years."

To the untrained observer, there appears to be little difference between the well-fed and restricted monkeys. "We don't see much difference in the behavior, comparing the control animals to the animals on caloric restriction," says Weindruch's colleague, Dr. Joe Kemnitz. "However, the restricted animals are more oriented to food and they show greater excitement at mealtime."

Among them is a lively, friendly monkey named Eeyore, after the donkey in A.A. Milne's *Winnie the Pooh.* Now seventeen years old, he has been on caloric restriction for eight years, nearly half his life. "He's very popular with the staff," says Kemnitz, "and very fit for his age."

Eeyore and his studymates are routinely anesthetized and x-rayed as part of the experiment. The scans of monkeys reveal extraordinary internal changes.

Compared to the well-fed monkeys, the calorie-restricted animals have much less fat but nearly as much muscle. They weigh on average one third less than the normal diet monkeys and have 10 percent body fat as opposed to 25 percent in the control group. Their bones are less dense, probably from bearing a lighter load, Kemnitz believes. If the diet is started at an early age, the bones tend to remain shorter and smaller in diameter.

The dieting monkeys are veritable small-scale versions of the fully fed group. "Everything is smaller," says Kemnitz.

The restricted monkeys, for example, had slightly lower body temperatures, by about half a degree. And the calorie-restricted monkeys were unquestionably healthier by every measure. Their metabolic rates were lower, pointing to more efficient use of energy. They have significantly lower levels of blood sugar or glucose, and this low glucose is a major factor in the health of all animals.

"The levels of glucose decrease in animals on caloric restriction," says Weindruch, "and so do insulin levels. But the insulin actually works better in the restricted animals to re-move glucose from the bloodstream and get it into cells where it can be used."

That is a significant finding, because rhesus monkeys, like their genetic human cousins, can and do get diabetes. In both cases, the body tends to produce less insulin as they grow older. As a result, cells take up less glucose, leaving more to percolate in the blood. This leads to a process called glyca-tion, wherein glucose molecules stick to proteins and other essential biochemical components. Like molasses in an engine, it gums up the machinery of the cell, making it per-form less efficiently and probably contributing to the aging process. Many of the secondary effects of diabetes, such as cataracts, are the result of this glycation process.

The calorie-restricted monkeys exhibit far fewer symp-toms of glycation and diabetes. "I think the most exciting find-ings currently relate to the fact that they're healthier, and most notably the fact that they are less prone to develop diabetes if they are on the restricted diet," says Weindruch. It's not just a happy failure to develop diabetes that marks the calorie-restricted monkeys. "They have favorable changes going on in the fats that circulate in their blood, like cholesterol and triglycerides. And their blood pressures are lower; all signs point toward improved health," concludes Weindruch.

The fully fed monkeys are not as lucky. One of them, named Moose, has developed diabetes and is on daily in-sulin shots. This is an unwelcome surprise for a middle-aged monkey because researchers believe diabetes accelerates the aging process by a third.

"So whatever it is that caloric restriction is doing, it's really retarding a very, very broad spectrum of age-related changes and creating animals which are extremely healthy and free of disease for very, very long periods of time for this species," says Weindruch. "And if we can mimic the basic mechanisms which are going on in the cells that are allowing these animals to live longer it would perhaps allow the same favorable result to occur for people as well."

Weindruch, like his mentor Dr. Walford, does not anticipate a worldwide tide of people suddenly restricting their intake to 1700 calories a day from the far more normal American diet of 2500 to 3500 calories a day. Rather, he envisions future development of a magic pill or two.

"One magic pill would allow us to eat less food and not be crazy about the situation. The other kind of magic pill would be the one or ones that mimic the most important effects going on in the cells, so that the basic mechanisms that are allowing these animals to live longer could be copied by drug treatment in animals and people eating normally," he says.

In another study at the National Institute on Aging, in Baltimore, Dr. George Roth, acting chief of the laboratory of cellular and molecular biology compared thirty calorie-restricted monkeys with thirty non-dieters that were also fed low fat foods. The monkeys receiving 30 percent fewer calories were also the beneficiaries of a number of changes generally associated with a lower risk of heart disease and stroke. Their blood levels of HDLs, the so-called "good" cholesterol, were higher, their triglycerides levels were lower, and the fat-laden potbellies displayed by the control group were absent. "Their biochemical markers for cardiovascular disease are moving in the right direction," said Roth.[26]

But it is the seeming ability of calorie restriction to prevent diabetes that most aging researchers find truly exciting. They know that diabetes hastens the aging process. Now, they ask, could blood sugar or glucose, the raw fuel that runs our bodies, hold a key to how we grow old? Biochemist Dr. Anthony Cerami, director of the Kenneth S. Warren Laboratories in Tarrytown, New York, believes there is a connection between glucose and the aging process. Through groundbreaking work with diabetes, he is now close to understanding one of the major reasons why we age.

"I became interested in the whole question of the complications of diabetes because my mother had diabetes," he explains. "And patients with diabetes have an accelerated form of aging. And so about twenty-five years ago, I started working on this and came up with the idea that it was glucose, which everyone thinks of as an energy source, actually had a very bad side to it, and could lead to the problems that are associated with the aging process."

What puzzled Cerami was the fact that people with diabetes, even when treated with insulin, still developed complications. "Most of those complications," he notes, "are the same as those non-diabetics get, but the diabetics get them at an earlier age. So, in effect, they are clinically aging at a faster rate. They get heart attacks, strokes, and cataracts earlier. They get a whole bunch of problems earlier. And we tried to understand that."

---

26. Grady, Denise, "Monkeys, Like Mice, Live Well and Prosper on Low-Calorie Diet," *The New York Times*, October 7, 1997.

What Cerami and his associates discovered was that the glucose in the blood of diabetics was reacting with hemoglobin, the protein that carries oxygen from the lungs into the cells of the body. As we age, blood sugar levels rise and the reaction increases, and more and more glucose binds to the hemoglobin, reducing its oxygen-carrying capability.

In the fossils of long-dead animals, Dr. Cerami sees the effects of glucose on old tissues and bones. In his office he points to the menacing-looking, huge, fanged skull of a Romanian cave bear that, he says, shows the process of glucose reacting with proteins quite well. "You can see that the teeth, as a result of being around for a hundred thousand years, have become quite yellow, and the bones are really quite brown as a result of the glucose reacting with proteins. We're undergoing this process all the time in our bodies, not quite to the level that this bear has, but if you look at the bones of an older person, they are in fact quite yellow. And this process is taking place in us as we're living."

Cerami uses simple kitchen chemistry to demonstrate exactly what happens when glucose reacts to proteins. He takes a chicken and pops it into the oven.

"Within a short period time," he says "you are going to see something you have seen many times, the chicken is going to develop a nice brown color as a result of being in the oven. This is a natural phenomenon that takes place not only at an elevated temperature, as we have taking place here in the oven, but also in the body at the body's temperature. Basically we are cooking very slowly over our lifetime."

It's quite a remarkable thesis. Food chemists, of course, have long known this process occurs when cooking and storing meats. "The chemistry," explains Cerami, "is in the reaction of glucose in the food with the proteins in the food. They rearrange and form those yellow-brown pigments that you see. If you've ever made a ham and put sugar on it, it turns brown faster because the sugar is basically driving the reaction, so it goes faster. You also probably know that if you cook a steak too long it gets tough. The reason is that these things also cross-link the proteins and that acts like a molecular glue sticking the proteins together so they can't move."

It took a long time before Cerami could convince the scientific community that this same process was happening inside our bodies. Like an overcooked piece of meat, we toughen over time. Our joints become stiff and our organs lose function, our bones and tissues turn yellow and brown. "If you look at the tissues of people as a function of age," says Cerami, "you can actually see the accumulation of these yellow-brown pigments."

Cerami has several slides of the lens of the eye that dramatically demonstrate his point. Taken from people killed in automobile accidents, the lenses range in age from those of a two-year-old to those of an eighty-year-old. The lens of the two-year-old is as clear as a pane of glass. That of a twenty-year-old is slightly tinged and grow progressively darker in the older lenses. Finally, the lens taken from the eighty-year-old is actually quite brown.

"You can do the same thing with teeth," Cerami says. "A young person's teeth are white and as people get older, their teeth get yellow because of the same reaction—sugars reacting with proteins. You can show a pathologist a bone and he can make a pretty good assessment of how old it is just by the color of the bone.

"Almost all of the major proteins that are involved—collagen, elastin, and others like that—accumulate these pigments as we get older. But the real problem with glucose isn't that your proteins are turning brown. The most important thing is that as a result of this, it makes everything stiff."

It happens because of the cross-linking of proteins, or glycation—the same biochemical event noted by Roy Walford and Rick Weindruch in their animal experiments.

In our blood vessels, protein chains are wrapped around balls of cholesterol. Glucose can anchor itself to the protein chain. It then undergoes several biochemical transformations and may eventually link to another part of the chain. Once cross-linked, cholesterol becomes harder to remove from the bloodstream.

But other glucose damage can occur. Blood-vessel walls are lined with strands of protein. If a cholesterol particle touches them, glucose can cross-link its protein chain to the wall. More cholesterol particles and glucose enter the tangle until the arteries become choked and clogged. The interior diameter of arterial open space closes, reducing the supply of blood to vital organs, causing heart attacks and strokes.

The end product of all this cross-linking is a protein glucose complex called Advanced Glyosylation End products, or AGE. The AGEs in turn cross-link among themselves, forming a sort of molecular glue. This causes the activity of the affected proteins to slow down and drastically reduces their flexibility. The result is a host of "opathies"—diseases familiar in both the elderly and the diabetic—neuropathy (nerve disease), retinopathy (eye disease), nephropathy (kidney disease), and atherosclerosis, the buildup of plaque in the coronary arteries causing heart disease.

Cerami has found that cross-linking is one of the major

causes of aging—in our skin, our lungs, our bones—
throughout our bodies. Now, after twenty years of investi-
gation, he believes he is close to finding a remedy. "Right
here we are involved in making a new compound that we
discovered that is really revolutionary in that it can break
the glucose cross-links that are responsible for the complications of aging."

Researchers once thought that cross-links could not be
broken—that they were permanent structures. But Cerami
and his colleague, Peter Ulrich, detected a telltale weakness.
"Everyone always thought that cross-links were very stable
but they are actually sitting there waiting to be broken," says
Ulrich. This was the clue they needed to develop a new drug.

"If you have two proteins that are cross-linked with a glucose molecule, this new class of compounds, breakers, that
we have, can come in and break that cross-link and smash it
apart, and allow the molecules to then separate in space so
they are no longer tied together," explains Cerami. "So things
that are stiff now will now become flexible again. All we have
to do now is just keep developing it and making sure that it's
OK. The drug has been successfully tested in laboratory animals, and now human trials are underway. If this new drug
works, it could reduce the stiffening of our joints and rejuvenate our heart and blood vessels."

Called Timagedine, the drug is specifically designed to
slow down the progression of diabetic complications. More
than 1200 people in the United States and Canada are par-
ticipating in clinical trials of Timagedine. The results thus
far are promising but more testing and fine-tuning are part
of the process.

"What I would like to see is seventy-, eighty-, and ninety-year-olds being able to function as well as sixty-year-olds, and if we could achieve that, I think we would certainly make the quality of life for people much better. I think that we now have an understanding of what's happening, and we should be able to achieve this goal, and I'm really very hopeful that we're going to be able to do it. I'm counting on it so much, because I want to be able to enjoy the fruits of this type of therapy."

Cerami has proved that glucose, the fuel we need to live, is slowly killing us. It is a double-edged sword that both gives life and takes it away. But something else essential to our bodies is also slowly destroying us.

At Southern Methodist University in Dallas, Dr. Raj Sohal is researching that other essential ingredient of life—oxygen. Sohal is doing uncommon research with the common housefly. Sohal's subjects are among the most annoying insects in most people's lives, and they are also among the most ideal subjects in which to study aging.

"We study houseflies because they have a short life span, and they age fast, and they breathe air just like humans do," he explains. "And we think that they age the same way as other air-breathing animals like humans." Flies, Sohal points out, are very enthusiastic fliers. "When flies undertake a flight," he says, "from a sitting state up, its rate of oxygen consumption increases by fifty to one hundred times."

To find out how oxygen affects aging, Sohal has an entire room devoted to houseflies. By restricting the motion of some of these flies, he can reduce their oxygen consumption. In the "fly room" the flies are confined in different containers. One group is stored in urine specimen jars—one fly per jar. Inside the jar, a cardboard maze divides the space. Flight under these conditions is not an option. The urine-jarred flies lead placid, sedentary lives. Others are confined in one-foot cubic cages—two-hundred flies per cage. The caged flies lead more normal housefly lives, flying around, buzzing, chasing, and interacting with each other.

"When we look at the life spans, the flies that have been raised in a bottle live about two to three times longer than the flies that have been kept in cages," says Sohal. "And this allows us to vary the rate of aging. The more active they are, the shorter their lives. So by simply preventing them from flying, the life span can be doubled or tripled. And these are the monks. They don't chase each other, they don't fly, and the food and water are here. They live a long time."

The monks live two to three times longer, Sohal has learned, because they use less oxygen. A flying fly consumes up to one hundred times more oxygen than a walking fly. And it's oxygen's role in manufacturing the body's energy that seems to make the flyers die sooner.

Any mechanism that increases oxygen consumption, Sohal discovered, will reduce the housefly's life span. Sex, for example, inevitably shortens the male's life. In this regard the male flies may be following the same path natural selection has laid out for Australia's marsupial mice, the antechinus (see Chapter Three). The problem for the male fly is that female flies mate only once in their lives. Male flies, however, are driven to mate constantly.

"In any population where there are relatively few females, the males are frantically looking for sexually receptive females," explains Sohal. "And this increases their activity and thus decreases their life span. For example, if instead of 200 male flies in the cage, I put 150 females and 50 male flies, those male flies live longer, because they fly less. There are sexually receptive females and they don't have to frantically look for a receptive one."

But alter the ratio of male to female the other way, and it's the female whose life is shortened. "If on the other hand, we have 175 males and 25 females, the life span of the females actually decrease. We think they are being chased too much by the males.

"In the case of flies any kind of experimental treatment that would affect their level of physical activity, enhance their rate of oxygen consumption, affects their life span. The more active they are, the shorter they live."

Sohal has found he can manipulate the rate of oxygen consumption by raising or lowering the temperature. Normal temperature in the fly room is 25 degrees centigrade. When Sohal changes the temperature to 18 degrees, the flies live twice as long. Elevating the temperature to 30 degrees shortens their life span by 70 to 80 percent.

What is it about oxygen, which is so essential to life, that also eats away our bodies with the rust of aging? It is a problem and process that began billions of years ago, when the first primordial cells were formed. The first, primitive, self-replicating cells were walled in by fatty membranes, envelopes that allowed them to organize into compact, efficient units that were protected from the churning primordial seas in which they floated. It was a time of great turbulence on the still cooling earth, and the tiny cells were to play a major role in changing the chemical composition of the gas envelope that covered it. The atmosphere, composed mostly of relatively inert nitrogen, was suddenly infused with a new, highly reactive gas—oxygen.

Over millions of years, the one-celled plants began to drift together, forming first clumps and then huge mats, hungry for energy. They found it through a chemical reaction called photosynthesis—using sunlight to draw hydrogen out of the water and converting it to energy. The by-product of all this chemical reactivity was oxygen, which the plants released into the air.

The oxygen was like a flame-thrower, burning through delicate cell membranes, searing proteins, cross-linking them into charred lumps, and tearing apart the most critical molecules of all, the DNA that programmed the cells. Untold billions of cells died, victims of their own lust for energy.

But natural selection favored a group of cells that had developed the ability to generate enzymes that could defuse the awful destructive power of oxygen and the even more destructive free radicals it formed. Free radicals are molecules that have been stripped of one of its normal complement of two electrons and are thus highly reactive. That means they career about inside the cells looking for another electron to pair up with. In the process, free radicals damage proteins, lipids, and DNA anywhere in the cells. The enzymes SODs, or superoxide dismutase, catalase, and glutathione peroxidase combined with the free radicals and turned them into water and less reactive forms of oxygen that could pass benignly through the cells.

This led the way to the formation of animal cells to use oxygen for energy. The result was an explosion of growth. The animal cells began to organize and develop into multicelled creatures that could use and defuse oxygen. From these beginnings, all creatures, including humans, evolved.

But it was a perilous trade-off, a delicate balancing act between the need for energy and the ravages of oxygen free radicals. Species with weak antioxidant defenses, like brilliant sparks, burned brightly but briefly. Their lives were short. Those better able to quench the destructive fires of oxygen—such as humans—lived longest.

And herein lies nature's ultimate paradox: the fires of life, using sugar as fuel and oxygen to burn it, create a buildup of by-products that create the ashes of aging. "Oxygen is a paradoxical substance that we use," Sohal says. "On the one hand, it gives us life. We cannot survive without oxygen for more than a few seconds. And in the long run, it is also very dangerous because its use necessarily involves the generation of radicals, which are slowly killing us. Living and dying are part of the same coin."

The thin line between life and death has always been a concern for Sohal. As a young boy in India he came down with polio. He turned to biology and the study of insects, allowing his mind to race when his body could not.

"Of course there are insects everywhere around in India," he says. "And it's hard to love those insects. But when I was an undergraduate student, I learned that insects are fantastic models for studying any problem in biochemistry or physiology."

In particular, Sohal found that insects were fantastic models for studying free radicals. With another fly, the fruit fly, he looked for deeper connections between oxygen damage and aging. He found them in the cell. Inside all animal cells are hundreds of structures called mitochondria. These are tiny intracellular structures that serve as the cell's power plants, where nutrients and oxygen are converted into adenosine triphosphate, or ATP, in the short hand of biology. ATP generates the energy for most cell processes, such as pumping ions across cell membranes, contracting muscle fibers, and building proteins. The entire cycle generates the fuel that powers the machinery of life.

Unfortunately the machinery in the mitochondria that produces ATP also generates the highly destructive oxygen free radicals. "The components of mitochondria—including the ATP-synthesizing machinery and the mitochondrial DNA that give rise to some of that machinery—are believed to be most vulnerable," writes Dr. Richard Weindruch. "Presumably they are at risk in part because they reside at or near the 'ground zero' site of free-radical generation and so are constantly bombarded by the oxidizing agents."[27]

The damage to the mitochondria is believed to jam the cycle, reducing production of ATP and increasing the output of free radicals. The process is like a doomsday machine— more free radicals flying about increases the destruction of mitochondrial components, reducing ATP production still further. Nor is the damage limited to the mitochondria. Free radicals escape into the cell proper further reducing its ability to function properly. "As cells become less efficient, so do the tissues and organs they compose, and the body itself becomes less able to cope with challenges to its stability," writes Weindruch.[28]

---

27. Weindruch, Richard, "Calorie Restriction and Aging," *Scientific American*, January 1996.
28. Weindruch, "Calorie Restriction and Aging."

Sohal and other researchers believe this free-radical damage is a major cause of aging. "The major finding that we have made in the flies is that the rate of free-radical generation increases during the aging of the flies and their tissues get progressively more damaged as the flies are aging," he says. "And what excites us about this is that the magnitude of the damage that takes place is sufficient to explain why these flies slow down, and it seems to explain a lot of the changes that are taking place here in the aging process."

Free radicals harm us despite the fact that our bodies have a natural defense system to fight off their damage. When an oxygen free radical flies off the assembly line a special enzyme can turn it into a less dangerous substance—hydrogen peroxide.

But when it leaks out of the mitochondrion membrane, and seeps into the cell's nucleus, hydrogen peroxide becomes less benign. There it can encounter an iron atom—creating the hydroxyl radical. This, the most dangerous free radical of all, destroys everything around it—including the DNA. But with luck hydrogen peroxide will instead encounter another protective enzyme, superoxide dismutase, that converts it into harmless water.

Sohal wondered if he could artificially strengthen this natural free radical–fighting system in his fruit flies. Could he create a genetically new superfly? First he isolated the gene responsible for producing the protective enzymes that make up the antioxidative system within the cell. Next, the gene's DNA was injected into fruit fly embryos.

"The hope is that these pieces of DNA would get inserted into the nuclei," explains Sohal, "and then the future flies would all contain extra copies of this gene in every cell. And they would then produce enzymes, and those enzymes would provide better protection against the free radicals."

The new batch of genetically engineered flies proved to be quite remarkable. "The most obvious difference between the genetically engineered fruit flies that were expressing these two extra genes was that they walked faster, they were friskier than the control flies. You could even tell the difference by just looking at them side by side. The flies that contained the extra copies [of the gene] were moving faster and their movement, even at old age, were friskier than the controls."

And, most remarkable of all, the flies with the genetically enhanced antioxidant system lived longer than the control group. In fact they lived 30 percent longer than the normal flies. It was a landmark achievement. Never before had scientists extended life by inserting genes into an organism.

"It was very, very exciting, and I knew that this is a fundamental discovery," says Sohal. "And whenever you make a breakthrough in science, which is quite rare, it is a moment to cherish.

"Of course the ultimate purpose of our research is to benefit man. Hopefully what we learn would help understand the basis of the aging process. If we understand the mechanisms of aging then it is possible that we can come up with some ways to intervene, to ameliorate the effects of aging."

Although not specifically the result of aging, there is one devastating disease, amyotrophic lateral sclerosis (ALS), or Lou Gehrig's disease, that has just been linked to a breakdown in the antioxidative process. In 1998, after five years of intensive searching, scientists at the University of Texas Medical Branch at Galveston (UTMB) discovered that a defective form of the SOD1 gene was partly responsible for causing the progressive nerve degeneration of Lou Gehrig's disease.

Lou Gehrig's disease, named after the legendary New York Yankee slugger whose baseball career it ended, is a progressive disease in which nerve cells that control muscle movement gradually deteriorate, causing eventual paralysis, loss of muscle and breathing function, and death. It normally hits people between the ages of twenty and fifty. Average life expectancy after diagnosis is two to five years. The hereditary form of the disease accounts for only about 10 percent of cases, with the rest arising from unknown, nonhereditary causes. Approximately thirty thousand Americans suffer from ALS. There is no treatment for the disease.

How a mutation in the SOD1 gene causes ALS has been a mystery, but scientists have speculated that the disease may arise because the defective enzyme can't clear away the dangerous free radicals. Without the protection offered by the normal protein, free radicals probably build up and degrade various body products, including the membranes and proteins that make up nerve cells.

The idea finds adherents among many neuroscientists because superoxide dismutase is found in higher levels in motor neurons, the nerve cells that control muscle movement, and are destroyed as ALS progresses. However, the idea never received strong experimental support, in part because it is technically very difficult to measure whether free-radical levels actually increase in live animals with ALS.

But the UTMB researchers were able to show that mice genetically engineered to carry a mutant form of the human

SOD1 gene had higher levels of free radicals than mice carrying the normal form of that gene. "With our evidence, the free-radical hypothesis for ALS is no longer just a theory," says Danxia Liu, an associate professor of neurology and human biological chemistry and genetics, who led the research team.

Liu and her colleagues also took tissue samples and measured levels of chemicals likely to be produced by free-radical damage, including products made from the breakdown of proteins, membrane lipids, and DNA. Those chemicals were present in higher levels in mice with mutant forms of the superoxide dismutase gene. Although the exact role of free radicals in the development of ALS remains to be determined, Liu believes the new findings are an important clue for researchers trying to figure out how ALS progresses.

"Maybe free radicals are the cause of the motor neuron deterioration, or maybe they are just part of a more complex process," Liu says. "But this evidence suggests that they are definitely involved in this disease."

Ultimately genetic therapy may prove to be the answer to Lou Gehrig's disease and many of the diseases of aging. But, since the insertion of antioxidant genes is not an option for humans yet, Dr. Raj Sohal suggests wine and vegetables.

"Wine," he explains, "has substances called poly-phenolic flavenoids and they are very good antioxidants. Ethanol itself is also an antioxidant, but these flavenoids are particularly good and they prevent oxidation of the lipids, which cause atherosclerosis. You've heard about the French paradox, the people in France drink a lot of wine and they also have fatty foods, lots of cheese and yet they're remarkably free of heart disease, especially as compared to Americans. The hypothesis is that it is due to the fact that they drink a lot of red wine and eat a lot of green vegetables."

Dr. Jeffrey Blumberg, assistant director of the Human Nutrition Center on Aging at Tufts University, is in enthusiastic agreement. "One of the elements to successful aging is to eat lots of fruits and vegetables. They are very rich in vitamins and minerals and what we call phyto chemicals. There are all sorts of ingredients in fruits and vegetables that seem to reduce our risk for cancer and heart disease. So fruits and vegetables are good for not only what they don't give you but also what they do give you. And we are just discovering now the nature of the thousands of different compounds in fruits and vegetables that seem to promote health."

In part that may be because they are full of free-radical fighters called antioxidants. The critical antioxidants are vitamins C and E—each protecting a different part of the cell.

Vitamin E resides in fatty cell membranes. When a free radical comes along, vitamin E traps and neutralizes it. Another free-radical scavenger is vitamin C, which floats freely inside the watery part of the cell. A free radical encountering vitamin C will also be deactivated.

Most vitamins were discovered between 1900 and 1950 and for most of that time were considered little more than a health fad. Scientists were skeptical about their benefits. Now they are taking them seriously. For the first time experimental studies are testing their promising claims. The science of vitamins is opening up a whole new era in how nutrition affects aging.

Every study ever undertaken has demonstrated the benefits of a high consumption of fruits and vegetables. These vitamin rich foods, especially vitamins C, E, and betacarotene, can boost immune function, reduce the risk of cancer and heart disease. But, will these foods and vitamin supplements extend life or simply make us healthier? "Even if antioxidant vitamins only block some age-related diseases and not the aging process itself," says Tufts Jeffrey Blumberg, "the advantage to increasing consumption is evident."

Vitamin E, for example, in its antioxidant guise, is particularly effective in heightening the immune response. "We've shown very nicely in clinical trials that as you get older your immune function declines, white bleed cells become less responsive so you're more vulnerable to infectious diseases and things like cancer. We have shown that in older people, when we've given them supplements of vitamin E, we boost their levels of immune responses to levels that makes them look thirty years younger," says Blumberg.

Vitamin C has dramatically reduced cataract formation in the elderly. "We've got nice data on the use of vitamin C supplements," notes Blumberg, "reducing by some 80 percent the prevalence of advanced cataracts. That's not exactly a terminal disease, the most commonly done surgical procedure in the United States is lens extractions, and the implications [are] not only for the quality of life we could offer these people, but also the health-care costs for doing all these surgeries could be reduced substantially."

Antioxidants might also delay or even prevent the development of those horrors of old age, Alzheimer's disease and dementia. A National Institute of Aging study of people with aging-related Alzheimer's disease found that those whose diets were supplemented with high doses of vitamin E experienced a delay of about seven months before reaching the next significant milestones in their illness: loss of the ability to perform the activities of daily living, moving to a nursing home, progression to severe dementia, and death.

The Basel [Switzerland] Longitudinal Study followed 442 Swiss men and women, ages sixty-five to ninety-two for twenty years. Those with high levels of antioxidant vitamins in their blood performed better in memory tests. "Disturbances in memory functions related to aging could be linked to increased oxidative stress with aging," said Dr. Hannes Staehelin, a professor of geriatrics at the University of Basel. "It's quite clear that neurons in the brain cells are challenged by free radicals and that the aging process itself is linked to free radicals. It appears that antioxidants actually protect the neurons from damage."[29]

The heart too will benefit from large amounts of vitamins. A recently published study of 80,082 female nurses who have reported on their diet, lifestyle, and health every two years for fourteen years, has shown that consumption of large amounts of folic acid and vitamin B_6 may sharply reduce the risk of heart attack. The Nurses Health Study, led by Dr. Eric B. Rimm of the Harvard School of Public Health in Boston, compared the amount of folic acid and vitamin B_6 in the diets of 658 women who suffered nonfatal heart attacks and 281 who had fatal heart attacks to those who had never suffered a heart attack.

Published in the February 1998 *Journal of the American Medical Association,* the study found a direct correlation between those consuming the highest levels and the lowest risk. Those women who averaged 400 micrograms of folic

_____

29. "Dementia Linked to Vitamin C and Betacarotene," *Australian Associated Press*, August 19, 1997.

acid and 3 milligrams of vitamin B₆ a day were 47 percent to 51 percent less likely to suffer a heart attack than those who consumed the least amount.

"We were surprised to see that for women with the highest intake of both vitamins in the diet, heart disease risk was almost cut in half, compared to women with low intake of both," said Rimm. "In fact, our findings suggest that to reduce risk of coronary heart disease, daily vitamin intake of folic acid and B₆ ought to be higher than current RDA [Recommended Daily Allowance]."

The results bolster a controversial theory proposed by Harvard pathologist Kilmer S. McCully. In 1969 he suggested that homocysteine, an amino acid found in the blood, might be as significant a risk factor as cholesterol. Homocysteine is formed when the body breaks down methionine, another amino acid found in food. Homocysteine then abrades blood vessel walls, priming them for a buildup of cholesterol deposits, with the inevitable narrowing of arteries greatly increasing the risk of heart attack.

After years of skepticism, McCully's theory is receiving more and more acceptance as more and more studies support the theory. They show that people with high blood levels of homocysteine are at a higher risk of heart attack. Other studies indicated that folic acid and B₆ reduced homocysteine levels in the blood. Now, the Nurses Health Study seems to confirm the relationship between homocysteine, heart attack, and the beneficial effect of vitamins.

For McCully, now at the Veterans Affairs Medical Center in Providence, Rhode Island, the new study was "strong evidence in support of the homocysteine theory.... It's quite impressive." The study also bolsters his belief that the sharp decrease in heart disease in the United States over the last few decades may be due in large part to people eating more fresh fruits and vegetables, thereby bolstering their diet with vitamin B$_6$ and folic acid.

"This is not the case that there's a new magic bullet out there," said Dr. Rimm, "but this suggests there is something to the 'eat five servings of fruits and vegetables a day.' It may be making small changes in our diets could go a long way toward reducing our heart attack risk."

It appears then that if we want to add healthy years to our lives, we had better listen to mother and eat our veggies. That and add supplemental vitamins until such time as we can be genetically re-engineered to manufacture our own antioxidants.

"There is no magic elixir for aging," says Dr. Blumberg. "It is everything we do combined together, but I can't think of a better way to start living a healthy life than to put lots of fruits and vegetables into your diet."

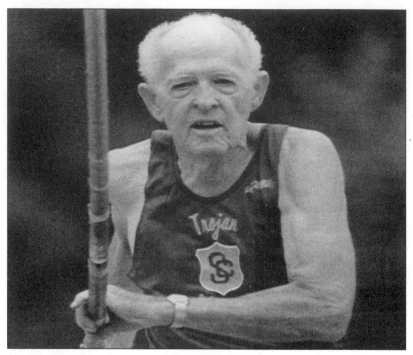

According to scientists, this octogenarian pole-vaulter soon will no longer be an exception to the kinds of activities practiced by the elderly.

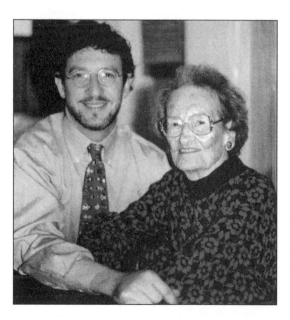

Harvard Medical School researcher and director of the New England Centenarian Study Thomas Perls, with 104-year-old Angeline Strandal, believes that centenarians have a genetic ability to remain healthy as they get older, and that we may soon be able to identify these genetic passwords.

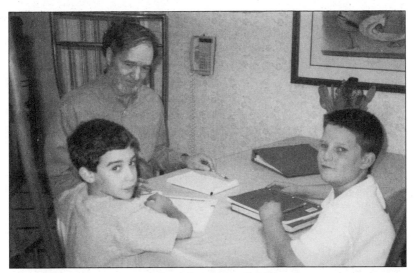

After years of study at the UCLA School of Medicine, physiologist Jared Diamond, pictured here at home with his sons, has concluded that the human's gradual ability to defend itself created less pressure to reproduce quickly and more investment in self-repair, promoting longer life spans.

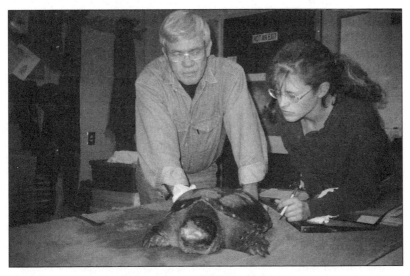

Whitfield Gibbons, professor of ecology at the University of Georgia, shown here with a colleague, has trapped almost 20,000 turtles along the Savannah River in the heart of South Carolina since 1968. When a creature is relatively safe—as the turtle is, thanks to its shell—it makes sense to repair itself year after year.

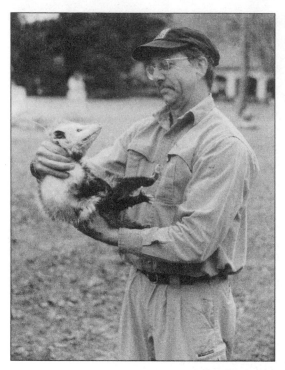

Steven Austad, professor of zoology at the University of Idaho, has found that opossums on a predator-free island off the coast of Georgia have a different genetic makeup and live 50 percent longer than their mainland-based counterparts who live with persistent stress.

Michael Rose, professor of evolutionary biology at the University of California at Irvine, has doubled the life span of the fruit fly. To Rose, these flies prove that human aging can be altered in ways that dramatically surpass current aging remedies.

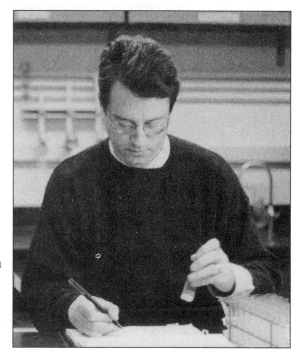

Professor of biology Thomas Johnson, right, with a member of his University of Colorado team, below, has doubled the life span of the nematode, a one-millimeter-long worm. The team has discovered that aging in the nematode is governed by "master genes," and hopes to discover the genes that affect humans in a similar way. The genetic mutations are studied under a powerful microscope and viewed on the monitor.

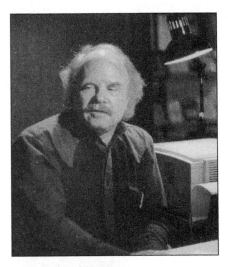

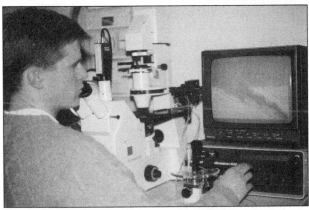

Seventy-four-year-old Roy Walford, right, a professor of pathology at the University of California at Los Angeles Medical School, is experimenting with caloric restriction—diets low in calories but high in nutrients. "Many alive today will live not only in the twenty-first century, but beyond it into the twenty-second century."

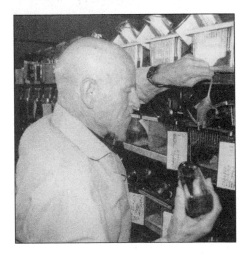

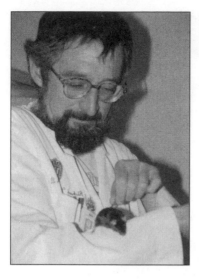

Rick Weindruch, professor at the University of Wisconsin Regional Primate Research Center in Madison, is conducting new work in caloric restriction on mice as well as rhesus monkeys, one step closer to applying the science to humans.

Raj Sohal, professor of biology at Southern Methodist University in Dallas, is studying the effects of oxygen free radicals. He has been working with houseflies for more than thirty years, and has found that by reducing their oxygen consumption, he can double or triple their life spans.

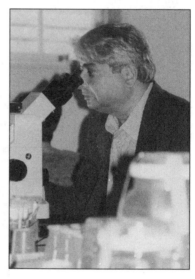

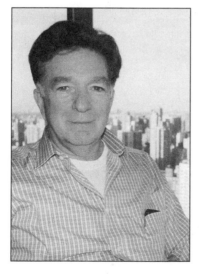

Anthony Cerami, a biochemist and director of the Kenneth S. Warren Laboratories in Tarrytown, New York, believes there is a connection between glucose and the aging process. Cerami has proved that glucose, the fuel we need to live, is slowly killing us.

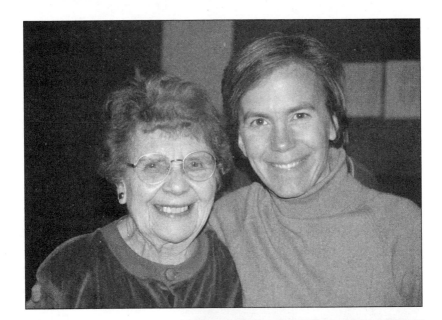

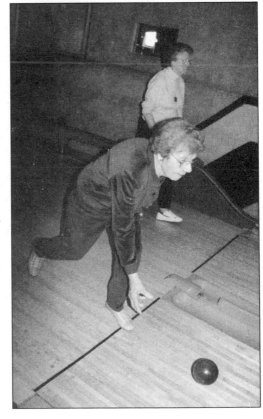

Miriam Nelson (on right, above), director of the Center of Physical Activity Programs and Policy at Tufts University's School of Nutrition Science and Policy and an assistant professor of nutrition, shattered an old medical assumption by discovering that age-related muscle loss can be reversed. When she started a strength-training program for elderly women, which included ninety-one-year-old Bernice Rice (on left above and seen here bowling), she discovered that bodies can build muscle at any age.

Judith Campisi, head of the Department of Cell and Molecular Biology at the Lawrence Berkeley National Laboratory in California, is studying the aging of cells. Most cells stop dividing at some point and become "senescent." Then some of them begin to malfunction, producing proteins that damage our tissues.

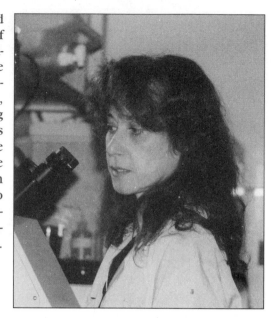

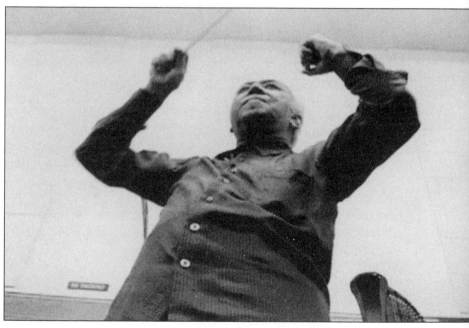

Symphony conductor Mehli Mehta, ninety-year-old father of Zubin Mehta and conductor emeritus of the American Youth Symphony in Los Angeles, is an example of an individual whose life contradicts the traditional view of aging as he continues to conduct all of his concerts from memory.

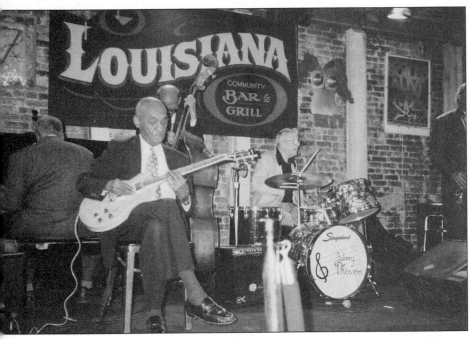

Harlem Jazz Legends guitarist Al Casey, age eighty-two, is another prime example of how extended lives may bring continued growth in careers, skills, and passion.

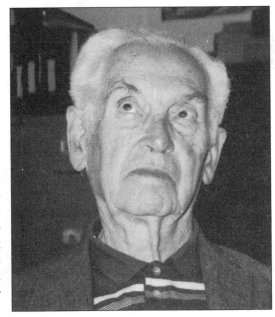

Ninety-four-year-old Ernst Mayr, professor emeritus of zoology at Harvard University, has trouble remembering some people's names, but is still very active in his scientific studies.

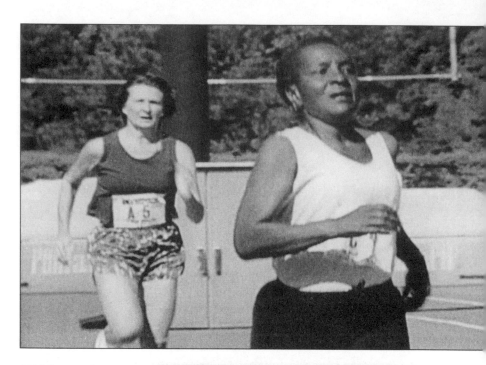

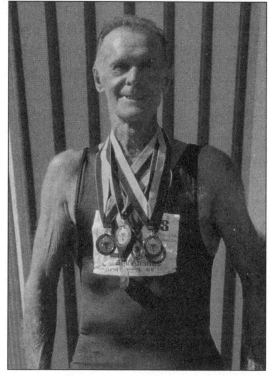

Middle-aged runners are currently staying healthy through exercise. In the not-too-distant future, record-breaking athletes may be fifty or sixty years old and look as if they are twenty-five. In fact, people will be fit and healthy until the very end of life, at ages of 150 or possibly 200. Remarkable older athletes, such as Senior Olympic gold medalist Jim Stooley, on right, will be much more common.

5   *Exercise and Hormones*

Eating your fruits and vegetables is a low-tech solution to living a longer, healthier life. Another low-tech solution is exercise. In Boston, Dr. Miriam Nelson, Associate Chief of the Human Physiology Laboratory at the Jean Mayer USDA Human Nutrition Research Center on Aging at Tufts University, believes that exercise is not only the key to staying healthy, it can also reverse an important part of the aging process.

She has been a maverick in her field—challenging age-old medical assumptions—and practices what she preaches. "I love to exercise," she says, "I always have ever since I was a little kid, and our family has always been really athletic but I think one of the interesting things being a scientist is seeing the amazing difference that exercise can make for people of all sorts of ages, even up to their nineties."

As proof she points to the exploits of master athletes, including a champion pole-vaulter and hurdler and track athletes in their seventies, eighties, and nineties.

"The first research that we ever did here at Tufts was actually to look at how master athletes compared to their sedentary age-matched counterparts," she says. "And what we saw without exception was that these master athletes were about twenty or thirty or forty years younger, biologically, than their sedentary counterparts. They had hearts and muscle strength and coordination, even though they were in their sixties and seventies, like that of someone in their twenties or thirties."

Most people, however, are not master athletes. Only one out of four Americans exercises. Children with seemingly limitless energy stores and boundless curiosity should be in a state of perpetual motion. The reality is that only a small percentage of American children are physically active on a daily basis. A shocking 22 percent are overweight.

Dr. Nelson ascribes the situation to the example set by parents. "I think it is because we as parents in general are out of shape and not physically active and overweight. Our children are just following in our footsteps, and so I think that we need to break this cycle and as families become more active so that our children will carry on that legacy."

Women, who are the focus of Dr. Nelson's research, are piling on the pounds and suffering from a host problems associated with obesity. "The reality is that 50 to 60 percent of middle-aged women, depending on which ethnic groups you're looking at, are overweight. And that's quite remarkable in that obesity is probably more due to a lack of physical activity than it is to overeating. We just don't expend calories because we're not physically active as a nation," says Nelson.

That problem is compounded by age. As we age, we gain body fat and lose muscle. At about age forty we begin to lose about a third of a pound of muscle every year. At the same time we gain that much or more body fat. In addition, we lose bone. For women who are smaller than men, the impact is even greater.

"We naturally have more body fat and less muscle," explains Nelson, "so we're losing at the same rate as men, but we're naturally going to be physically weaker than men. That's why it's critically important for a woman to take care of her muscles and her bones so that she can remain strong for a long period of time."

The loss of strength becomes an increasing handicap as we age. "Muscle strength becomes a limiting factor in our lives as we get older," explains Nelson. "So that getting out of a chair, which requires muscle strength, becomes a problem. So that carrying groceries is difficult. Even walking around the block, which you think of as a cardiovascular workout, actually needs muscle strength to do as well. So that many of the activities of daily living need a lot of muscle strength in order for us to continue doing them easily."

Knowing this, Nelson began a bold experiment trying to reverse the muscle loss typical of old age. She and her colleagues started a strength-training program for elderly women. Some in her field said it would never work. They thought it was risky because lifting weights might damage old, flaccid muscles and hurt frail bones. But Nelson's hunch was right—it worked.

"When our research first came out in the late eighties and early nineties most of the medical community were really astounded that these women can rebuild muscle that they have lost as they have gotten older. In just about two months or so we can see the reversal of the sort of normal age-related losses of muscle. We have seen up to three or four pounds of muscle gain with that much fat loss so it's just a complete reverse of what you normally think of with the aging process."

Nelson had shattered an old medical assumption. She had discovered that you can build muscle at any age. This was welcome news for ninety-one-and-a-half-year-old Bernice Rice. A feisty, diminutive woman, Rice was not about to be slowed down by injury. "Three years ago I broke my ankle and the doctor said I could plan on walking with at least a cane or maybe a walker for the rest of my life," she recalled while bowling. Her response was hardly typical of the doctor's patients. "I just replied, 'Those are fighting words.'"

After joining Nelson's program, Bernice's ankle healed completely. She developed new muscle, denser bones, and physically tested twenty years younger than her actual age.

"It is never too late to start exercising, as we've seen with Bernice, who is ninety-one. We even have people in their later nineties and early hundreds, and we see the difference that it can make. Strengthening exercises and endurance types of exercising can make a real difference in how these people feel about themselves and how they age," says Nelson.

The research at Tufts has shown positive benefits in virtually every area of health. Women who have undergone the strength-training program have reported they are not only stronger, but also have more confidence and self-esteem. They sleep better and are emotionally stronger, ready to take on new challenges they would never have thought of tackling before.

Strength training also seems to ally one of the greatest fears of old age—falling—because it builds stronger bones. "While we are challenging our muscles," says Nelson, "the muscles in turn challenge the bone. What we've seen in the year-long study with just two days a week of strength training is increasing bone density, both at the hip and the spine, and also improvements in muscle strength, muscle mass, and dynamic balance. If a woman is strong and has good balance she's going to be more resistant to a fall. And if we can keep her from falling she's not going to break her hip. If she happens to fall, her bones are going to be denser so that she's less likely to break a hip. So both the balance, the muscle strength, and the improved bones really put a woman at a reduced risk of having a fracture as she gets older."

Aging muscles might one day get a boost from genetic therapy. Scientists at the University of Pennsylvania Medical Center in Philadelphia have developed a gene therapy treatment that permanently blocks the age-related loss of muscle size and strength in mice. Mice, like humans and indeed all mammals, lose up to a third of their muscle mass and power with age. In humans, the result is an advancing weakness in the elderly that can lead to unsteadiness and impaired mobility, increased susceptibility to falls and injury, and joint stress and degeneration.

Even in young adult mice, the new treatment increased muscle strength by a dramatic 15 percent over untreated muscle. But in older mice, the improvement was even more remarkable: The researchers documented a 27 percent increase in strength over untreated muscle in these mice—fully restoring their strength to what it was in young adulthood.

The technique suggests human therapies that could reverse the feebleness associated with old age or counter the muscle-wasting effects of muscular dystrophies and related diseases. The results of the experimental study were published in the December 22, 1998 issue of the *Proceedings of the National Academy of Sciences.* "Our results show that it may be possible to preserve muscle size and strength in old age using this approach," says H. Lee Sweeney, Ph.D., a professor of physiology and senior investigator on the study. "We're now looking to see whether the technique might also be used to increase muscle strength in diseases such as muscular dystrophy."

The new treatment utilized the ability of some viruses to integrate their genetic material into the cells they infect. Their choice was an adeno-associated virus, or AAV, known to be highly efficient at introducing its genes into target cells. They then stripped the AAV of its own disease-causing—and immune-system provoking—genes. The stripped virus was then reloaded with a normally occurring gene called insulin-like growth factor, IGF-1, a hormone critical in the process of muscle repair. They also fed in a muscle-specific promoter to drive high production levels of the growth factor. The researchers then injected the engineered virus into the muscles of the mice.

Under normal circumstances, damaged muscles release quantities of IGF-1 as an activation signal to neighboring cells known as satellite cells. Satellite cells are muscle stem cells—progenitor cells—that become functional muscle cells after activation and then migrate into the muscle to repair it.

The researchers theorized that age-related muscle loss might be the result of a declining efficiency in the satellite-cell activation process due to a decreased IGF-1 signaling capability with age on the part of muscles in need of repair. The hope was that the virus delivered genes would order high levels of IGF-1 production in aging muscle, thereby stimulating more effective repair and regeneration by the satellite cells. And it worked.

Until such time as muscle and strength-enhancing gene therapy becomes readily available, exercise remains the only game in town. But you don't have to work out at a championship level to benefit from exercise. Research shows that if you walk even an hour every day, you increase your life span by two years. And two recent studies published in the *Journal of the American Medical Association* even offer hope to couch potatoes. The first, by the Cooper Institute of Aerobics Research in Dallas, followed 235 sedentary men and women, ages thirty-five to sixty, who were divided into two groups and monitored over two years. One group, the gym rats, spent twenty to sixty minutes vigorously exercising—swimming, biking, or doing some other aerobic exercise—up to five days a week. The other group, the couch potatoes, incorporated thirty minutes a day of the "lifestyle" exercise. These included such mundane tasks as raking leaves, climbing stairs, or even pushing a grocery cart through the supermarket.

The findings surprised and even deflated some exercise gurus. At the end of six months, both groups had similar—and significant—improvements in cholesterol ratios, blood pressure, and body fat percentages. The lifestyle group did, however, have to exercise three times longer than the gym rats to burn the same amount of calories.

The second study, which followed forty obese women, had similar results. This is good news for people who normally do not exercise. Researchers have found they are more likely to stick to a regimen of doing everyday activities than keep up with a daily gym routine.

"We can all start a program, and most people do in January," said Dr. Andrea Dunn, a Cooper Institute researcher and lead author of that study. "And by February, 50 percent of those people have stopped. If we don't develop approaches that are easier for people, we'll continue to have the public health problem that we have at the moment." The studies are among the first clinical trials to find that moderate exercise is beneficial for the one in four Americans who spend most of their time sitting and incubating heart disease.

Even more deflating to the proponents of vigorous exercise were the results of a Mayo Clinic study that suggested that merely moving around or fidgeting could help people stay trim. Before one sinks into the depths of the couch content that an occasional wiggle or scratch will keep one fit, bear in mind that the researchers involved in these studies are not recommending that people stop working out at the gym. Nor do they say that a lunchtime walk here and a set of stairs there will be enough to substantially improve cardiovascular fitness.

"It has to be a little more structured than that," said Dr. Ross Andersen of Johns Hopkins University. "It's not just haphazardly doing ten minutes on Monday and ten minutes on Tuesday. And it has to be done at a purposeful pace."[30]

---

30. "Daily Activity Can Improve Fitness," *Associated Press*, January 27, 1999.

There seems little doubt that regular exercise does pay off. Still another study reports that women who exercise four hours a week cut their risk of breast cancer by more than a third. It is also thought that moderate exercise may boost the human free radical–fighting system keeping pace with the extra oxygen damage that comes from working out.

When John Glenn's soared into space at age seventy-seven, in October 1998, he not only offered a raft of new data on exercise and aging in a weightless environment, but, according Wayne Osness, exercise physiologist at the University of Kansas, may have inspired some older adults to begin a fitness program. "I think John will teach us a lot about the quality of life with his bout in space," states Osness, who researches fitness in people of all ages. "Glenn had rigorous physical training as a young man and has been in training all of his adult life. But older adults who haven't trained as Glenn has shouldn't assume they can't regain some flexibility and stamina."

Osness says that despite the differences between a seventy-seven-year-old astronaut and a seventy-seven-year-old nursing-home resident unable to get out of bed and walk to the bathroom, both can benefit from an exercise program matched to their level of fitness. "The good news is as a result of our research, we can we can turn fitness levels around for people who have lost the flexibility to get out of bed. They won't be able to run any races, but many can get out of bed and go to the bathroom and back. Or they can leave the house and sit in a car and go for a ride. These are major changes in the quality of life for older adults.

"Exercise activates physiological processes necessary for flexibility, which is important to our quality of life, whether we want to pull a lever in a spacecraft or reach for something on the top shelf in a kitchen cabinet."

Muscle tissue atrophies in space because the force of gravity is gone. "Our bodies are trained in gravity. Gravity dictates the way we sit or stand. Anyone who has been bedridden for six weeks experiences tissue atrophy similar to what astronauts experience," Osness notes.

Surprisingly, Osness found that older adults, in their seventies or eighties or older, are comparatively easy to motivate to improve their fitness. "Teenagers find it difficult to look ahead," he says. "Generally they are in good shape and have fewer self-image problems. Middle-aged adults find they can do less than they could, their body structure is changing and they have a desire to do something about it."[31]

In Miriam Nelson's view it is the single most important thing anyone can do to help themselves. "Exercise," declares the Tufts professor, "is probably the most important thing that an older person can do to remain vital and independent, especially because it affects their muscles, it affects their bones, it affects their mental acuity, and, in fact, if we could package exercise up in a pill form it would be the single most widely prescribed medication in the world because it does so much for everybody."

Some people think that a magic pill may already be here. At the National Institute on Aging in Baltimore, Maryland, scientists are studying the role of hormones in later life. Hormones are tiny chemical messengers continually secreted into the blood stream by the endocrine glands. The purpose

---

31. "No Age Limit On Exercising Options," *University of Kansas Report*, October 23, 1998.

is to regulate the activities of vital organs. The word "hormone" comes from the Greek word *hormaein,* which means to set in motion or spur on. Hormones stimulate a host of life-supporting processes throughout the body to maintain health, growth, healing and repair. Unfortunately, most hormone levels decrease naturally as we age. Among those declining hormones that are thought to be a factor in aging is human growth hormone or HGH.

Produced by the pituitary gland, HGH is a small molecule similar to insulin. Secreted into the bloodstream in short pulses during sleep, it remains in the circulation for only a few minutes, making it extremely difficult to measure.

During adolescence when the body grows at its most rapid rate, HGH production is very high, hence the name growth hormone. But, even when growth has ceased, HGH continues to pulse into the blood, albeit at lower levels, to maintain a healthy body. "Tissue repair, healing, cell replacement, organ integrity, bone strength, brain function, enzyme production, integrity of hair, nails, and skin all require the ongoing availability of adequate growth hormone. After age twenty, growth hormone production falls progressively at an average rate of about 14 percent per decade. By age sixty, it is not uncommon to measure a growth hormone loss of 75 percent or more. Physical decline with age correlates directly with decreased secretion of growth hormone by the pituitary gland," wrote Drs. Elmer Cranton and James Frackelton, in the magazine *Alternative Medicine.*[32]

"Approximately every three years 90 percent of the cells

---

32. Cranton, Elmer M., M.D. and Frackelton, James P., M.D., "Growth Hormone to Reverse Aging," *Alternative Medicine,* June 1995.

in the human body are made anew," they noted. "The body is composed of more than 100 trillion cells which are continuously dying and being replaced. Only in the brain and nervous system are the original cells (neurons) retained, but proteins are continuously being made in the brain to store memories of each new experience. Learning, memory, and intelligence all depend on adequate growth hormone. As growth hormone falls with age, functions of all vital organs decrease."

Part of the problem is the tendency of older people to become increasingly sedentary. "Physical activity, particularly aerobic exercise, sets off the release of growth hormone in people of all ages," says Dr. Marc Blackman, chief of endocrinology at the Johns Hopkins Bayview Medical Center, in Baltimore, Maryland. "Sedentary people who become physically active frequently have bursts of growth hormone release."

All this has not escaped the notice of researchers. "It has recently become clear that growth hormone is important for grown-ups," says Dr. Mitchell Harmon of the NIA. "We used to think it made kids grow from being small to being normal height. It turns out that when you lose growth hormone for one reason or another, you lose muscle, you gain body fat, your whole quality of life changes. And when the growth hormone is replaced people feel better."

Replacing growth hormone was an inordinately difficult task until fairly recently. Harvested from the pituitary glands of cadavers, HGH was used almost exclusively to treat dwarfism in children. But in the late 1980s biotech companies learned to synthesize the molecule and that opened the way for scientists to study its effects on aging. Among the first researchers to study the effects of HGH on the elderly was a team led by the late Dr. Daniel Rudman at the Medical College of Wisconsin in Milwaukee. In 1990 he published the results of a study conducted on men sixty-one to eighty-one years of age. All showed very low levels of HGH in their blood. The men were divided into two groups. The first group of twelve men received injections of HGH three times a week, while a control group of nine men received no treatment. At the end of six months, the results were quite startling.

"The administration of human growth hormone for six months in group one was accompanied by an 8.8 percent increase in lean body mass, a 14.4 percent decrease in adipose-tissue mass, and a 1.6 percent increase in average lumbar vertebral bone density," reported Rudman. "Skin thickness increased by 7.1 percent. In group two there was no significant change in lean body mass, the mass of adipose tissue, skin thickness, or bone density during treatment."

Rudman's conclusion: "The findings in this study are consistent with the hypothesis that the decrease in lean body mass, the increase in adipose-tissue mass, and the thinning of the skin that occur in older men are caused in part by reduced activity of the growth hormone . . . and can be restored in part by the administration of human growth hormone. The effects of human growth hormone on lean body mass and adipose-tissue mass were equivalent in magnitude to the changes incurred during ten to twenty years of aging."[33]

In other words, the men given regular injections of growth

---

33. Rudman, Daniel, M.D., et al., "Effects of Human Growth Hormone in Men Over 60 Years Old," *New England Journal of Medicine*, July 5, 1990.

hormone experienced an astonishing reversal of from ten to twenty years of the aging process. They increased muscle, shed body fat, had stronger bones, and found new vitality.

Based on Rudman's results, the National Institute of Aging provided $5 million to fund several studies at nine major university medical centers. One of the projects is headed by Drs. Harmon and Blackman at Johns Hopkins. It is a typically double-blind study in which one group receives the HGH and the other a placebo, and no one knows who is getting what. The results are not yet in, but the researchers already see changes in several people in the study group.

"We don't know what are our subjects are getting," says Harmon. "But a number of our subjects have said that they are sexier, that they feel stronger, that their *joie de vivre* has improved, that they feel more energetic, that they want to go places, and that they had a kind of energy that they didn't have before we started treating them."

At another center, the University of Washington in Seattle, another method of delivering HGH is being explored by Drs. Robert S. Schwartz and George Merriam. GHRH, or growth hormone-releasing hormone, the brain chemical that triggers the pituitary gland to release growth hormone into the bloodstream, is used.

"Our preliminary findings include significant changes in body composition—a decrease in body fat and increase in lean body mass due to the hormone and in some cases to exercise—and a complete absence of side effects," Dr. Merriam said.

"Treating a person with the brain's releasing factor for growth hormone instead of with growth hormone itself," he explained, "should better mimic the body's natural pulsed output of the hormone and diminish possible side effects, like swelling of tissues and aggravation of diabetes and congestive heart failure."[34]

Other hormones have also been found that can seemingly affect the aging process. One called DHEA, for dehydroepiandrosterone, is produced in the adrenal cortex, the gland that sits atop the kidney. DHEA is a best-selling, health-food store steroid and a favorite pick-me-up of fitness buffs. Among the least understood of the endocrine hormones, its major attraction to scientists is as a biomarker for the aging process. From youth through the early adult years, the adrenals pump out DHEA in steadily rising quantities. Then, as the body continues to age production declines. By the age of eighty, people have 80 to 90 percent less DHEA in their blood than they did at the age of twenty-five.

At the NIA's Arizona Center on Aging, a team led by Dr. Mark Lane used DHEA as a marker to trace the aging rate in calorically restricted monkeys. Levels of the hormone were found to be higher in the calorically restricted monkeys.

"DHEA levels are of great interest to us," said Lane, "not because we believe that DHEA is the fountain of youth, but rather because it gives us a very good marker to measure the rates of aging in control versus calorically restricted monkeys. It is important to distinguish between levels of DHEA that occur naturally in the body and decline with age and levels that are seen in people who pop DHEA pills to pharmacologically raise their natural levels in hope of extending their lives."

---

34. Brody, Jane, "Restoring Ebbing Hormones May Slow Aging," *The New York Times*, July 18, 1995.

Lane doesn't know whether the artificially higher levels of DHEA are benefiting the pill poppers. "Controlled clinical trials are needed before this question can be answered," says Lane.[35]

A few such trials have been conducted. In June 1995, Dr. Samuel S.C. Yen of the University of California, San Diego, reported on DHEA administered in doses of just large enough to replace age-related losses, to more than fifty men and women over the age of fifty.

"People felt better," said Dr. Yen, "their muscle mass increased, blood levels of insulin-like growth factor, which keeps cells healthy, also increased. In men, an increase in interleukin-2 and natural killer cells indicated activation of the immune function."

It all sounds marvelous and a number of people, including physicians, are using and touting the benefits of DHEA as a sort of Methuselah pill. On the Internet DHEA is promoted as the "Mother of Hormones" and the "amazing anti-aging pill."

But a one-year follow-up study by Arlene Morales, a researcher at UCSD, using ten milligrams of DHEA, reported no increase in well-being. Lean body mass did increase and men, but not women, lost fat and improved their knee strength.

Still another early 1986 study generated remarkable results. Also at the University of California, San Diego, an epidemiologist named Elizabeth Barrett-Conner examined the blood levels of DHEA of 143 middle-aged and elderly men who had been followed for twelve years. Those with high

---

35. "Two New Studies Suggest that Caloric Restriction in Monkeys May Extend Their Life and Health," *NIH Report*, October 2, 1997.

levels in their blood suffered half as many cases of heart disease as the men with low DHEA levels.

"The results were so incredible that I didn't believe them at first," Barrett-Conner says. "So I went back and pulled ninety-nine more blood samples. They showed the same thing."[36]

But five years later, Barrett-Conner did a larger, follow-up study and found that high DHEA levels lowered the risk of heart disease in men by only 20 percent, about the same as other studies had shown. "Every five years a new wonder drug comes along," she said at a 1995 meeting held by the New York Academy of Sciences on DHEA. "Well, I don't think DHEA is the wonder drug the people at the meeting seemed to think it is."[37] The bottom line then on DHEA seems to be a question mark. Magic elixirs are perhaps just that, fairy-tale remedies that work in stories but not real life. Still, there are no dearth of hormones and people touting them.

Melatonin, sold for years as a dietary supplement, is now being hyped as an anti-aging hormone. Produced in the center of the brain by the pea-sized pineal gland, melatonin keeps the body's internal clock in sync with rhythms of night and day. Production of melatonin is stimulated by darkness and inhibited by bright light. It is an essential monitor of changes in the length of the day and changing seasons. This becomes a critical signal for the reproductive systems of many seasonal breeding mammals. Through its actions on other hormones, it mediates bio-clock functions such as when sheep and other animals breed, when peo-

---

36. Bilger, Burkhard, "Forever Young," *The Sciences*, September/October 1995.

37. Bilger, "Forever Young."

ple sleep, when birds migrate, and when dogs shed their coats.

Like other putative anti-aging hormones, melatonin production declines with age. But it was not until a series of controversial studies in mice by Italian endocrinologist Walter Pierpaoli, of the Biancalana-Masera Foundation for the Aged in Ancona, Italy, and William Regelson of the Medical College of Virginia that melatonin became a darling of the health-food, anti-aging crowd. The two researchers spiked the mice's drinking water with melatonin and reported they lived an average of six months longer, were more vigorous and sexually active, and had better immune systems than the control group of mice drinking unsupplemented water.

In a second set of experiments in 1994, Pierpaoli and Regelson transplanted pineal glands from young mice into old ones. The transplanted mice were also rejuvenated and lived longer than a control group. The two researchers concluded that melatonin produced by the young, transplanted pineal glands was the agent responsible. They described the results of their studies in a book *The Melatonin Miracle*.[38]

Unfortunately their conclusions ran afoul of one of science's cardinal rules—the results of any experiment must be reproducible by other scientists. They have not been. The first problem was that the strain of mice used by Pierpaoli and Regelson were genetically incapable of producing melatonin. In other strains of mice, melatonin supplements induced lethal tumors, thus shortening rather than lengthening life.

---

38. Pierpaoli, Walter, M.D.,Ph.D., and Regelson, William, M.D., with Colman, Carol, *The Melatonin Miracle*, Simon & Schuster, New York, 1995.

Melatonin does, however, appear to enhance the immune function, and may provide an antioxidant effect to reduce cell damage. But as Amnon Brzezinski of Israel's Hebrew University reported in the *New England Journal of Medicine,* "There are no data supporting an anti-aging effect in humans."[39]

The raging hormones of youth and sex, testosterone and estrogen, are another group of biochemical messengers that are being investigated for their longevity stretching effects. Estrogen, the female hormone, does not normally fall into the anti-aging category, but estrogen replacement therapy has been proven to reduce the frequency of heart disease, stroke, and death from all causes among post-menopausal women. Dr. Bruce Ettinger studied the medical histories of 454 women born between 1900 and 1915 and compared the health of those who received estrogen replacement therapy and those who did not. A little more than half the group, 232, used the replacement therapy for at least a year beginning in 1969. All were members of the Kaiser Permanente Medical Care Program in Oakland, California. The study, reported in the September 1997 issue of *Journal of Obstetrics and Gynecology,* found that women on the estrogen pill had a death rate 46 percent lower than their counterparts who did not take the pill.

"The overall benefit of long-term estrogen use is large and positive," Ettinger wrote. "Women who use this relatively inexpensive drug can substantially reduce their overall risk of dying prematurely."

Testosterone, the male sex hormone, has a far more para-

---

39. "Can Hormones Stop Aging?," *Washington Post,* February 24, 1998.

doxical effect. In some instances it has been found to shorten rather than lengthen life. In others, it has been seen as a restorer of youth and vigor to aging males. Manufactured in the testes, the hormone is responsible for male facial and body hair patterns, deep voices, and, of course, macho swagger. Aging men, who are victims of diminishing libidos and softening muscles and increasing deposits of fat, are increasingly looking to testosterone for a hormonal pick-me-up.

A 1992 study by Dr. Joyce Tenover at the Emory University Medical School in Atlanta, Georgia, gave thirteen elderly men testosterone for three months and a placebo for three months. While taking the hormone, the men increased muscle mass and excreted less bone mineral. Their cholesterol levels dropped and their libido picked up.

Other small studies have produced similar results, including a personal experiment by Dr. Norman Orentriech. Nominally a New York dermatologist, he and his staff of sixty nurses and doctors transplant hair plugs into balding pates (a technique he invented), smooth out wrinkles, and perform other wonders to create the silky skins of the rich and famous.

But Orentriech is extraordinarily well-versed in endocrinology and biology and has been the lead researcher on a number of studies of DHEA for the NIA. His interest is also buoyed by a continuing personal study in the use of hormones—taking DHEA and testosterone on a regular basis.

"I've been taking topical testosterone myself for fifteen years," he told author Gail Sheehy in 1996 for an article in *Vanity Fair*. "I was almost sixty. My morning erections were down. Libido was down. My beard was getting soft. My waist developed a girdle of fat. I was feeling tired and down. When I measured my blood, my androgen levels were down around 300."

"All classic symptoms of male menopause," added author Sheehy, editorially.

After Orentriech began applying a testosterone-releasing patch, he noticed a distinct improvement. "My sexual appetite and competency is back to where it was when I was around forty. And testosterone is an antidepressant beyond words.... I cannot tell you how many vital men I've made."[40]

Lurking in the background, however, is the very real fear that even small doses of testosterone could spark the growth of prostate tumors. Testosterone also speeds up the production of red cells, thickening the blood and thereby increasing the risk of stroke. Given the boost to the libido, many men are apparently willing to take the risks, but it is doubtful that testosterone will actually extend their lives. In fact, it may reduce longevity.

In one of the few studies ever done on castrated men, who for obvious reasons lose their ability to manufacture testosterone, the unfortunate eunuchs lived longer than a matched group of intact men. The appalling experiment was conducted from the late nineteenth and well into the twentieth century to control the violent behavior of male inmates in a Kansas institution for the mentally retarded.

"Experience with domestic animals and later with eunuchs apparently encouraged the belief that castrated males tend to be more tractable than intact males," noted James Hamilton and Gordon Mestler of the Department of Anatomy at the State University of New York College of Medicine. The two researchers authored a historical study of the practice and its effect on the longevity of the inmate population.

---

40. Sheehy, Gail, "Endless Youth," *Vanity Fair*, June 1996.

"The main part of this study was of mentally retarded white Ss [subjects]; 735 intact males, 883 intact females, and 297 eunuchs.... Survival was significantly better in eunuchs than in intact males, beginning at twenty-five years of age and continuing throughout life. The median (the estimated average duration of life) was 69.3 years in eunuchs, 55.7 years in intact males.

"Eunuchs also significantly outlived intact females.... This is considered to be evidence that orchiectomy [castration] prolonged life, since it seems impossible to select males who would outlive females in the absence of orchiectomy."

Since testosterone is released in great floods after puberty, the authors also compared the age at which castration occurred to longevity. "Males castrated at eight to fourteen years of age (before sexual maturation) were longer lived than males castrated at twenty to thirty-nine years of age (after sexual maturation). Castration between eight and thirty-nine years of age was associated with reduction of 0.28 years in age at death for every year of delay before orchiectomy. That progressive lowering of age at castration was associated with progressive lengthening of life after forty years of age was considered to be further evidence of an effect of orchiectomy upon survival."[41]

It is hardly a recommended means of achieving longer life.

Hormones notwithstanding, something happens throughout life to the organs, tissues, and cells that make up our bodies. They suffer from insults both external and internal that

41. Hamilton, James B., Ph.D., and Mestler, Gordon E., "Mortality and Survival: Comparison of Eunuchs with Intact Men and Women in a Mentally Retarded Population," *Journal of Gerontology*, 1969, Vol. 24, No.4.

cause them to function less efficiently and to die off. In short , they age, or, as the biologists say, they senesce. But when and where does senescence begin? Does it occur in the body as a whole, in individual organs, or in the cells? In 1961, Leonard Hayflick, at the time a professor of medical microbiology at Stanford University, set out to answer those questions.

Growing fetal cells in cultures, he watched as they divided and redivided. With no need to keep a larger organism alive, the cells doubled and redoubled like some magical multiply-ing machine. Then, after about fifty divisions the cycle stopped. The cells altered their behavior, consuming less food, repairing their membranes less frequently and less effi-ciently. In short, they showed all the signs of cellular aging.

Then, Hayflick repeated the experiment, but this time with cells from a seventy-year-old. These older cells also divided and redivided, but this time they stopped after about twenty or thirty doublings. Cellular aging had begun much earlier, in all probability because the cells themselves were older than those in the original experiment.

"What we were seeing," said Hayflick, now professor of anatomy at the University of California, San Francisco, "was the concept of cellular aging, growing older in the micro-cosm of a petri dish."

Growing older, but not necessarily decrepit. Hayflick esti-mated the amount of cells that could be produced from one cell, if they all were saved, on the order of twenty million tons. "This mass of cells," he noted in his book *How and Why We Age*,[42] "is far more than anyone's body would need in a

_____

42. Hayflick, Leonard, *How and Why We Age,* Ballantine Books, New York, 1994.

lifetime. Apparently nature has endowed us with cells that are mortal, but that have sufficient division and functional capacity to satisfy our needs for far more than our maximum life span of 115 years."

And what was true for human cells seemed to hold true for all species. Normal cells from long-lived animals divided many more times before they died than did cells from shorter-lived species. Newborn mice live for only 3 years, but their cells divide about 15 times. The cells of newborn chickens, which live for 12 years, divided about 25 times, while the cells of a Galapagos turtle, which lives for 175 years, divided about 110 times. "There seems to be a direct relationship between species life span and the number of population doublings that its cultured cells will undergo," concluded Hayflick.

That does not mean that aging and death are a lockstep reaction to cell division. "I do not believe that people age or die because their cells stop dividing. I think that the range of changes that occur in cells before they lose their capacity to divide or function affects the whole body in such a way as to make it more vulnerable to the diseases of old age," says Hayflick.

But why should nature so over-engineer the organism? Cells that can live for more than a hundred years are not a very efficient investment in a body that will only last seventy years. Scientists wrestled with that conundrum for quite a while until they discovered the method in nature's seeming profligacy.

Dr. Judith Campisi, head of the Department of Cell and Molecular Biology at the Lawrence Berkeley National Lab, believes it may be a means of preventing older cells from turning cancerous. Campisi was another of the ten scientists attending the March 1999 conference assessing the progress made in the science of aging.

"We think the reason why we evolved this mechanism of stopping cell division after a certain number of divisions is as a tumor-suppressant mechanism."

But old cells don't simply stop dividing and fade away, rather, many remain alive and become what biologists call "senescent." Campisi describes the sequence of events as follows:

Actually, three things happen when a cell undergoes senescence. The first thing is it stops dividing. If you think about it, anything that limits cell division is potentially a means of limiting cancer. And, in fact we think the genes that limit proliferation are important genes for limiting cancer.

But two other things happen when cells undergo senescence. The first is the cells lose their sensitivity to dying. Normal cells have an intrinsic genetic program that tells them when to die. If they're in the wrong place at the wrong time, or if they are damaged, they have a suicide program that basically allows that cell to quietly go away. Senescent cells lose that ability. They become much more resistant to signals that would normally tell a cell to die.

The third thing that happens when cells senesce is they begin to function abnormally. We think that the fact that senescent cells do not function normally, coupled to the fact that they don't die, may be why they may contribute to the aging of organisms. So what happens is the longer you live, the greater the chance you have of accumulating senescent cells that do not have the good grace to die, and certainly don't function normally.

All this adds up to a breakdown of the tissues and organs of the body. "There is some evidence that cellular senescence may contribute to the decline in tissue function that occurs with aging. It may be one of the contributing factors to aging," says Campisi. She has also learned that older people have more senescent cells than younger people. These malfunctioning cells may be why with old age our wounds heal more slowly, our skin wrinkles, and our ability to fight disease weakens. With senescent cells, Campisi has found a fundamental new process of aging.

"The theory of cell senescence and aging," she says, "is based on the fact that the abnormal function of senescent cells enables them to secrete molecules that can act at large distances within the tissue. So as we age and as senescent cells accumulate they produce molecules that eventually destroy the integrity and the function of the tissue."

Among those molecules is an enzyme called collagenase, which is produced by fibroblasts, the cells that make up human skin. The fibroblasts float in a sea of collagen, a protein that gives skin its flexibility and thickness. Each fibroblast is like a tire-repair kit, manufacturing collagenase to patch and repair burned or cut skin. The collagenase breaks down the damaged collagen and sweeps it away. Fibroblasts then divide in sufficient numbers to replace the damaged cells and pump out new collagen to return the skin to its original healthy form. But, when more and more fibroblasts become senescent, the repair process breaks down. "The cell seems to undergo a kind of derangement," says Campisi. "Instead of using collagenase selectively to clear away damage and spending most of their time pumping out collagen, the senescent cells start to pump out a large amount of collagenase, which eats away at the healthy collagen and almost stop pumping out collagen altogether."

The dividing and then senescing fibroblasts are a text-book example of what has come to be known as the "Hayflick limit." Leonard Hayflick's original seminal work alerted scientists to the seemingly unalterable rhythm that governed cellular division. It seemed reasonable then to assume that cells also aged in the body, winding down to the relentless beat of a ticking clock that measured off a finite time to live. Suddenly, the goal of aging research became a search for that ticking clock. If it could be found and, even more important, reset, longer living cells might give rise to longer living human beings.

The clock appears to be a string of seemingly nonsense DNA tips at the ends of each chromosome. Scientists have known about these tips since the 1930s, when they first discovered fragments of noncoding DNA—that is, DNA that does not give rise to proteins—at the ends of each chromosome. These tips, which have been likened to the plastic shells that cap the ends of shoelaces, are called telomeres, a combination of the Greek words for "end" and "part."

It was an intriguing finding, but the DNA that comprised the telomeres seemed to be so much biobabble, an arrangement of bases without seeming coherence or purpose. Then, in the 1970s, geneticist Barbara McClintock at the Cold Spring Harbor Laboratory on New York's Long Island, while working on corn, noticed that broken chromosomes were extremely unstable. Something, she hypothesized, must therefore protect normal chromosomes to keep them from malfunctioning.

That something was the telomere, and research into its

mysteries moved from corn to pond-water-dwelling protozoa, from the East Coast to the West Coast. At the University
of California, Berkeley, Dr. Elizabeth Blackburn and Dr.
Carol Greider, who was then a graduate student, began
studying the chromosomes of one-celled protozoa and
yeast cells in 1985. These creatures with thousands of tiny
chromosomes, compared to the mere forty-six pair in humans, provided countless telomeres that could be isolated
for study. They and other researchers soon learned that each
time a cell divides, the telomeres at the ends of the chromosomes are shortened. In mammalian cells the telomeres
eventually become so short the cell can no longer divide
and either dies or senesces.

But in their model one-celled systems, the cells continued
to divide, the telomere tips seemingly in inexhaustible supply. In 1987, Blackburn and Greider found the reason; an
enzyme called telomerase that acted as a rubber stamp, continually reprinting the proper DNA sequence onto the ends
of the telomere tips. Human cells also have the gene that produces telomerase, but in most normal cells it is permanently
switched off. But it is active in egg and sperm cells, where it
maintains the telomeres at youthful length. Telomerase is
also active in many cancer cells, which grow uncontrollably
far beyond the Hayflick limit, by somehow managing to
switch the gene on.

"The moment telomerase was discovered," said Leonard
Hayflick, "it was clear that for immortal cells at least, this was
a way to circumvent the inevitability of aging and dying."[43]

The telomerase gene, however, was quite elusive and it

---

43. "Can We Stay Young," *Time*, November 25, 1996.

was not until 1997 that a group headed by Nobel laureate Dr. Thomas Cech at the University of Colorado discovered the gene in another pond-dwelling creature called *Euplotes aediculatus*. Geron Corp., a biotechnology company in Menlo Park, California, founded primarily to explore the mysteries and doubtless commercial potential of the "telomere hypothesis," agreed to license the rights to the gene. But it was far from a human-ready, usable gene. It was, in fact, as the gene in a minute, simple, pond creature about as far removed from humans as it was possible to get on the evolutionary scale. Still the tree of evolution encompasses all life on earth, and somewhere Cech and his colleagues knew there had to be a human DNA counterpart. Sure enough, after months of searching the constantly expanding DNA data banks created by the human genome project, they found it, a fragment of human DNA whose sequence matched part of the *Euplotes* gene.

With it Cech was able to tweeze out from human cells the gene that makes the core of the telomerase enzyme. Geron scientists cloned the gene, as did a group from the University of Texas Southwestern Medical Center in Dallas. Both teams set up an experiment to coax normal cells into living far beyond the fifty-division Hayflick limit.

They inserted the gene into cultures of two different types of test-tube grown, middle-aged human cells whose telomerase-making gene was permanently switched off. The gene-treated cells in both laboratories quickly built their telomeres back to a youthful length. The control group of untreated cells kept on dividing until they all died. The telomerase-treated cells continued to double and re-double, with no signs of stopping.

The scientists see the immediate prospects as an aid in treating injuries and diseases rather than adding a century or two to human life. "It will now allow us to take a person's own cells, manipulate and rejuvenate them and give them back to the same patient," says Dr. Jerry Shay of the University of Texas Southwestern Medical Center. "The rejuvenated cells could help grow new skin for burn victims and in diseases caused by the failure of aging cells to divide, such as macular degeneration."

Will telomerase enable us to repeal the Hayflick limit and rejuvenate the entire body? There are too many imponderables for that question to be answered right now. Cells in vitro may age quite differently than people. And not all the cells in the body divide throughout life. Once fetal development is complete, most cells stop dividing. Only the cells that make up tissues and fluids that get a lot of wear and tear, such as the skin, blood, and stomach lining, continue to divide. And no one is certain whether those wear-and-tear tissues grow old and stop dividing when their telomeres run out. If they do, then telomerase might enable them to continue to divide and stay young.

Unfortunately telomerase may be the ultimate paradox. The system, as Dr. Campisi pointed out, has more than likely evolved, at least in humans, as a means of keeping cells from turning cancerous. Thus medically upping the division limit may weaken one of the body's inherent defenses against cancerous growths.

Dr. Robert Weinberg, a leading expert on cancer genetics at the Massachusetts Institute of Technology, believes there are enough telomeres in the cells to enable us to live to be two hundred. The limit on the human life span is diseases, especially cancer, and the shortening of the telomeres is the means nature uses to prevent the development of incipient cancer cells.

"If you put telomerase into all our cells, maybe they could live longer," Weinberg says, "but on balance it would be a very bad thing because it would no longer prevent those cells from growing without limits and, in the end, malignancy is the greatest threat to human longevity."

Still, it may be possible to switch telomerase genes on and off for specific periods of time, creating just enough telomeres to rejuvenate the cell, but not enough to turn it cancerous.

That prospect has gotten considerably brighter since the announcement by Geron at the end of December 1998 that the cells given the telomerase gene the previous January were still dividing without any sign of uncontrolled or cancerous growth. The Geron team, led by Choy-Pik Chiu, says its laboratory cultures of immortalized cells have doubled more than two hundred times—that's about four times as many divisions normal cells make, with their anti-cancer genes still in good order.

The Wright-Shay team at the University of Texas Southwestern Medical Center in Dallas said their altered cells had gone through 280 doublings, also without any sign of the random growth patterns typical of cancer cells.

This confirms the idea that the cells will "provide therapeutic opportunities for age-related diseases," the Geron scientists assert. But the company's plan is not to give patients cells with permanently activated telomerase, if it can avoid doing so. Rather, the hope is to develop drugs that will switch on telomerase temporarily, just long enough for it to rebuild the telomeres back to their youthful length.

"The responsible approach in the therapeutic development of telomerase is not to constitutively activate the enzyme but to control its regulation," Dr. Calvin Harley, Geron's chief scientific officer said.

Asked if Geron had yet developed drugs to switch the telomerase gene on and off, Harley said, "We have some data," but he added that the company's research is focused on understanding cells with permanently activated telomerase.[44]

Whether that understanding will lead to greatly extended, human life spans remains to be learned. For now, it seems safe to say that with the discovery of telomerase and the genes that control its manufacture, the Hayflick limits on aging have been lifted. How well we progress on that and other fronts will determine the future course of human longevity.

---

44. Wade, Nicholas, "So Far, So Good for 'Immortal' Cells," *The New York Times,* December 29, 1998.

6 Mastering the Mind

The traditional view of aging holds that after sixty people are past their intellectual prime; they should settle down and progressively withdraw from the challenges of the world. But some of the world's most creative people are old people. Indeed, civilization has been enriched immeasurably by artists, writers, and scientists such as Pablo Picasso, Georgia O'Keefe, Grandma Moses, Albert Einstein, Giuseppe Verdi, Robert Frost, and many, many others who all continued to be creative and productive to the end of their long lives.

They and the millions of sixty-year-old-plus people who continue to lead productive, creative satisfying lives constitute the central mystery that confounds aging research today. That is, given that most people are intellectually and physically sharp in their twenties and thirties, why in their seventies do they vary so greatly in mental ability?

Diseases, such as Alzheimer's (see Chapter Seven) account for some of the intellectual deterioration in the elderly. But, even for old people without disease, the variation in how well our minds work is enormous. Scientists agree that genes account for half of the difference at most, so what determines the rest?

How, for example, do we explain people like world famous and still working biologist Ernest Mayr, ninety-three, or the Harlem Jazz Legends, a band with four members in their eighties? Or George Burns, who until his death just before celebrating his one hundredth birthday was still performing before adoring audiences on stage, in the movies, and on television? Then there is ninety-year-old Mehli Mehta who conducts the American Youth Symphony as he has done for the past thirty-three years. Rather than retire and settle down, he spends his time shaping up the musicians of the twenty-first century. At eighty-nine, former chess-master Oscar Shapiro still travels all over America playing tournaments against opponents less than half his age.

Until recently, the view among scientists was, apart from a few unusual cases like these, mental decline with age was to be expected. One reason is that the brain becomes less adaptable with age. In the beginning, early in life, our brains are amazingly adaptable. Young children can learn a new language in months. In our twenties, our brains are at their peak. We know a lot and our brains work fast. And then, so the theory went, things go into decline. The brain loses the ability to change.

But a growing body of research is beginning to challenge this notion. A fair amount of it is the work of neuroscientists Marian Diamond at the University of California, Berkeley, and Arnold Scheibel, at the University of California, Los Angeles. Now in their seventies, the husband-and-wife team have spent much of their lives trying to understand what the brain can and cannot do as it ages. When they started out attitudes were very negative. Diamond says, "I can remember as a little girl being told that by forty I'd be going downhill. Well, I felt so good at forty, and then at fifty I felt good, and at sixty I felt good, at seventy I felt good. So you continue, I think the brain can decide its own destiny."

That destiny is determined in the billions of neurons—the key cells that comprise most of the mass of the brain. But the initial complement of neurons we have at birth must serve for a lifetime. With only a few exceptions, nerve cells do not grow back.

"We know there are neurons, nervous-derived cells in the olfactory system, that are continuously redeveloping during life," explains Scheibel. "There are cells in the hippocampus indentate which are parts of the old brain, concerned with memory, where you have slow, steady replication right through life. Marian's group has confirmed that. Those probably are the only ones, though, that are likely to do it. Otherwise, at birth what you have is what you're going to get. As a matter of fact, you're going to lose a very large complement of those in the first six months or year, year and a half of life. And so you have a focusing down to what I guess the nervous system considers the bare essentials of what we need."

Within that needful context, the neurons perform quite remarkably. "They do very special things," says Scheibel. "And there's probably a very good reason for not introducing hordes of new cells into the matrix of the cortex, because in a sense, the memories that we develop, the impressions we have and that are going to stay, are based on a certain kind of circuitry."

Indiscriminately adding whole new elements would essentially destroy the old circuits and create new ones. The fear is the existing bed of memories layered into the old circuits would be wiped out by the introduction of new circuitry.

Although there is a finite limit to the number of neurons we possess, they enhance their power by continually seeking out and making connections with other neurons, forming a dense web of interconnecting cells.

"A neuron," explains Professor Scheibel, "essentially matures by growing branches. The branches, or dendrites, are extensions of itself out into this space around it. This becomes the surface area on which connections, we call them synapses, are made."

The synapse, Greek for "clasp together," is where one neuron, or brain cell, talks to another. Incoming signals pass down the branches gathering together in the cell body where their information is processed and finally sent out as a signal along a long nerve fiber, the axon, which sends signals to the surface of other neurons. A single neuron can communicate with hundreds of thousands of others, forming a complex network of branches to store and process ideas. The number of synapses that link cells together varies greatly. Some cells may have as few as one or two thousand. In some parts of the brain there may be as many as 250,000 synapses on a single cell, each one receiving a signal or input. The greater the density of synapses, the greater the capacity for learning.

"The period of apparent maximal ease of learning seems to coincide with the period when there is the largest density of synapses per unit volume," notes Scheibel. "This is some time between the age of three or four and maybe six, seven, eight, nine, maybe even ten.

"So there's a very close correlation [with cognition]. And after that, as the number of synapses begins to taper off (and that's absolutely normal after ten), obviously individuals still learn very well, but the facility with which learning occurs changes.

"And you see this very clearly in language. Until about ten, the individual can learn virtually any language and bring it in, accent-free. After that, there is a little more trouble. It is seldom that the other second or third languages are unaccented. And even more interestingly, if you measure either with the new visualization techniques (such as PET or functional MRI) or actually measure when you're in on the living brain (in neurological surgical procedures, you can show that the brain area which is involved with the primary language is smaller than the brain area with the secondary and tertiary languages), if they were learned after this critical period. So that it really takes more cortex, bearing fewer synapses per unit volume area, to pick up the same kind of thing."

The end result is an extremely adaptive system that responds to stimuli by increasing the number of synapses to increase the ability to learn.

"We can show with our rats going into enriched environments, where several rats are living together in a large cage and having input, we can change those nerve cells measurably in four days," says Diamond. "Those are statistically significant differences."

"If you look at a microscopic level," adds Scheibel, "you can actually see changes beginning to occur on those surfaces of the dendrites within thirty seconds of the accession of a brand new input. It can occur that quickly."

Diamond and Scheibel's work has laid to rest one of the great misconceptions of twentieth-century neurobiology—that the older we got, the more brain cells we lost.

"Cell loss was the great bugaboo of neurologists and neuroscientists in the middle of the twentieth century. And we know now from a number of studies, such as Marian's, that in the healthy human brain, there is very, very little neuronal loss. As a matter of fact, the maximal cell loss we're ever going to suffer occurs around the perinatal period. And unless we are ill, we should never see anything like that again. Perhaps the best protection against cell loss is the active, refreshing life that one tries to live right through to the very end.

"But, in fact, changes do occur that are age-related in the brain. And one that everybody has validated is that we compute more slowly. We process more slowly. But that can also be an advantage, because in the extra time it takes us to make a decision, we're actually able to bring in far more perceptions and memories, and give a better-judged output. Perhaps you can call it wisdom."

Marian Diamond puts it more succinctly. "I would say that 'use it or lose it' came from our work. I remember at a cocktail party saying that for the first time to somebody. And they were really shocked that the brain could change at all. And so we've been speaking about this for over thirty years, and many people still don't believe that the brain will change positively with experience."

But it will, and that positive change is essential to growing old successfully. Indeed, if the thirty-odd years of work by Marian Diamond and Arthur Schiebel have proven anything it is that we must never lose our curiosity, our interest in the world around us and our desire to learn.

"Stimulation in general, by keeping curious, asking questions, wanting to learn for a lifetime, is essential," says Diamond. "But having the knowledge that your brain *can* change positively with aging helps tremendously. But we just say keeping curiosity, newness, and challenge. Not just taking the easy route. Taking something that is difficult. Maybe trying piano lessons later on. It is exceedingly difficult. But accept it, work hard at it, and enjoy the fruits of your labor when you're successful.

"Novelty is important. And that's why I think, as people travel, they've learned on their own that to take a trip, you have a lot of new planning, you have new geography, you have new currency. Everything you do when you're traveling is new and challenging. I think it's very healthy, but I think older people are recognizing this, and more and more are trying to fit it into their schedules."

Getting old, inevitably means retirement. In most western countries the retirement age is sixty-five.

"One of the great trends of aging in this country, given the wealth and privilege that's available," says Stanford University neurobiologist Dr. Robert Sapolsky, "which has gone down the drain, is 'what a great thing to stop working at age sixty-five!' Just halt everything dead at that point. And people have realized that's just a disaster for an awful lot of folks. But the other extreme of you just keep working in exactly the same way until you die in your proverbial boots, that's nobody's idea of pleasure in a lot of cases either.

"What people are realizing is the ideal thing is you gradually taper off over time. What's the tapering off about? There's a very realistic recognition of: what aspects of one's occupational expertise might simply be impossible at age seventy versus age fifty? What aspects are least rewarding? What aspects are least likely to work when you've slowed down a bit and when you're relying a bit more on older knowledge rather than new knowledge? That sort of thing. The sort of accurate assessment around the time things are tapering off, as to what are the parts that work well for you, and which parts do you have to realistically let go of?, that winds up being the work profile that I think is most associated with successful aging. Not the work yourself to death, and certainly not the at age sixty-five your work life and often your self-definition is dead."

In fact, there is no rationale for working for approximately forty or forty-five years and then suddenly stopping at an arbitrary age. But, ever since Otto Bismarck introduced the idea of retirement at age sixty-five in nineteenth-century Germany, that's when most people retire. Bismarck, while aspiring to win the office of chancellor of Prussia, observed that all his rivals in the government were sixty-five or older. Cleverly, so the story goes, he managed to have legislation passed forcing the retirement of all public servants sixty-five or older. Apocryphal or not, Bismarck did rise to power, united Germany under Prussian rule, fought and won two major European wars, and as a legacy, among other things, institutionalized the idea of retirement at age sixty-five throughout the industrial world.

It was a bad idea, at least in so far as keeping our brains stimulated and healthy.

"It certainly seems to go entirely counter to the research," says Scheibel. "I think there's a general feeling that many people don't really enjoy what they do, and so retirement is a wonderful excuse for stopping doing what you didn't like. But all of modern neurobiology tells us that this is precisely the wrong direction because, as Marian's work has shown, and as our work with humans has shown, dendrites retract a lot more easily than they grow. And as soon as you retire, unless you go to something that is absolutely new and different and equally challenging, hopefully more so, your [dendrites] are going to begin to retract. As you retract, your computational power decreases, too.

"It seems to me that when you finally decide that it's time to stop what you're doing, you should have in mind some very exciting things that you want to do next. And again, as Marian says, newness, unusualness is the key here. That which is new is difficult. That is what precisely challenges a part of the brain, an old part called the reticular formation, and it responds to newness, and it stimulates not only brain activity but brain growth. And that's what we're trying to achieve for the older person."

The pioneering work of Marian Diamond and Arthur Schiebel has helped to overturn a great deal of conventional wisdom. But many neuroscientists have clung stubbornly to the idea that it was impossible to teach old rats new tricks, especially when they'd spent their lives languishing in a cage. But at the Beckman Institute for Advanced Science and Technology at the University of Illinois, William T. Greenough is in fact teaching old rats new tricks, and increasing the size of their brains at the same time.

"A rat in a cage is kind of like what it would be to spend your whole life living in your own bedroom. We've referred to them as, 'cage potatoes,'" he says.

But what happens if a cage potato is given a change of scenery? Greenough wanted to find out. "Basically we wanted to replicate something of the natural environment for a mature animal, and turn the animal from a 'Wonder Bread' rat into a kind of normal, wild rat, and then see what happened in the animal's brain."

To do this, Greenough set up what he calls a Disney Land for rats. In a large cage he placed a group of rats and scattered toys throughout. The toys were changed on a daily basis.

"It's socially enriched," he points out. "There are lots of individual animals that the others can interact with. And it's very, very physically enriched or complicated or complex, providing new things to learn about, new things to explore, new things to understand."

The effects were dramatic. Within a few days of entering the enriched environment major changes had taken place in the rats' brains. Dendrites sprouted wildly, forming many new synaptic connections. And new blood vessels formed to bring extra blood to the rats' now more active brains.

It was a significant phenomenon. "The brain is interesting relative to the other organs of the body in the sense that it always essentially runs on empty," notes Greenough. "It doesn't store carbohydrate. It doesn't store oxygen. And hence it's dependent moment to moment on a good blood supply of both oxygen and carbohydrate. So if there's a higher level of demand, really the only way to accommodate this is to increase blood flow."

Like Diamond before him, Greenough found older rats' brains were significantly boosted, although they changed less rapidly than the brains of young rats. "First," he says, "the nerve cells or neurons differed. The neurons had more synaptic connections between cells, and more of the dendrites and axons that gave rise to these communicating connections. Connections basically constitute the wiring diagram of the brain, the processing hardware. And we think (although the proof still needs to come) that additional connections are actually associated with additional performance capacities, additional memory.

"The other thing we found is that the vasculature, the blood supply, was hypertrophied [enlarged] in the animals that grew up in the complex environment. They actually had a higher density of blood vessels, a higher number of capillaries per nerve cell."

The changes were rapid, over about three to four weeks, and were age dependent. "If a young animal goes into the complex environment, there's a near doubling of the number of blood vessels per nerve cell," says Greenough. "If a mature adult goes into the complex environment, there's an increase of somewhere between 15 and 25 percent."

The results were fascinating. But Greenough still had to answer the question: Was it exercise or was it the intellectual stimulation in the environment that was responsible? To do that he devised an experiment that separated the two components. One group of animals had an exercise wheel and with it they could exercise to their heart's content. A second group of animals learned a series of complicated motor skills but with relatively little physical exercise. This group was dubbed the acrobats. As a control a third group of cage potatoes was also included. Like human couch potatoes they had very little exercise and very little opportunity for learning.

After three months, the animals were sacrificed and their brains examined. Under the electron microscope, Greenough counted synapses, the junctions where one neuron talks to another, and the blood vessels that supplied the cells. The results were surprising.

"The animals that were in a basically dull environment, but did have the opportunity to exercise, actually did not differ from our cage potatoes in the number of synapses. But they increased selectively in the density of blood vessels to blood flow," says Greenough. "That is, the blood flow in particular was increased in these animals, but there was no detectable change in the number of synapses.

"What we found in the acrobats, the animals that learned new tasks with minimal exercise, is that the number of synapses increased. It actually embellished the wiring diagram of the brain. But the blood flow was not different from what we found in the animals that were left in boring, empty cages."

Scientists now accept that these experiments prove the brains of older rats are changeable. They change rapidly in response to environmental demands and opportunities. Enriching the environment enriches the brain.

Marian Diamond and Arthur Scheibel are convinced what's true for rats is true for humans. The key to good cognitive function, at any age, they believe, is novelty.

"There is a part of the brain which is built to detect novelty and alerts the rest of the brain," says Scheibel. "And with that alerting comes new dendritic growth, new circuits, and so forth."

With this in mind, these still active researchers are doing all they can to stimulate their own neurons. "We took up sculpting, which was something we hadn't done before," says Marian Diamond. "We know someday we want to try carving in marble. Right now we're just playing with clay. But that's down the line for something new. And we're doing piano again and Arnie's starting his violin. And taking up new sports."

The message is simple. A healthy brain needs continual stimulation—both physical and mental. A healthy brain needs new challenges. For at any age the brain can respond. It's not just a question of staying smart. Scientists examining brains of the deceased have found that, in general, brains with a large number of connections seem to help their owners.

Brains with higher numbers of synapses not only tend to have higher cognitive capacity but also appear to give resistance to the clinical symptoms of diseases like Alzheimer's. (See Chapter 7.)

For some successful agers, novelty is a way of life. At ninety-three, biologist Ernst Mayr lives in an intellectual Magic Kingdom. The ruling passion of his long life has been intellectual curiosity. The mental stimulation that results may well be responsible for his good health and acuity at the age of ninety-three.

"I always had a tremendous breadth of interest," he says. "I was interested in everything, I always wanted to know everything, read everything, and that included not just science but literature, the arts. I'm still very active. I'm writing small papers. I'm writing reviews. I answer an enormous amount of correspondence. And I'm working on two books."

At ninety, Mehli Mehta is the principal conductor of the American Youth Symphony in Los Angeles. He thinks the passionate all-encompassing world of music, especially conducting, has kept him young. "Conducting," he says, "is one of the most physically tiring things in the world. We not only concentrate, and think of the music and remember the music and all that. But we have to impart it to a hundred boys and girls or men and women who are in the orchestra. A good conductor uses this arm, the right arm, for the tempo and for the rhythms and all that, and the left arm for the expression. So both arms are working together. The chest is working, lungs are working, the brain is working, everything is working together except the legs. And even the legs. Just as we keep our body in good shape by exercising, you have to exercise your memory also. And therefore every concert throughout the season, a whole season, I do from memory. Thank God my memory is still in good shape."

Oscar Shapiro is a former chess master. At eighty-nine he believes the key to aging well lies in balancing challenge and fun. "I've improved year after year, I'm playing stronger players all the time," he notes. "Chess program on the computer, I play against it. And that helps a little, keeping me in practice. And my theory is you have to submerge your ego. You must not be afraid to lose. Many players, they just quit for fear of losing. They take it so seriously."

Scientists have tried to discover what successful agers like these have in common. Success, they found, seems to depend mainly on four things. First, intellectual enrichment is good for the brain. So educated people who continue learning life long, like the enriched rats, in general age well. Second, plenty of exercise ensures the brain is supplied with blood. A third characteristic is health: people who maintain good lung function and avoid cardiovascular disease in general age well. And finally something no lab rat has: a sense of control. Champion agers tend to have a realistic idea of what they can and cannot do. If these factors go some way toward explaining why some people age so well, they are only part of the story. These findings have been repeated and supported elsewhere, including a landmark Harvard study. (See Chapter Seven.)

Even the most successful of agers has losses. Scientists studying the aging brain have to account for these as well. For Mehli Mehta getting older has meant working harder to maintain a certain level of accomplishment.

"Of course, the older you get the more you have to practice. I've never heard of a great one who's playing after eighty-five. They play at home, of course, they play for their friends, they play chamber music. But to play at recitals and concertos and all that, fingers simply don't work. Fortunately for us conductors, we don't have to play the notes. Thank God. Maybe I was quicker and I was sharper when I was younger, but I'm much more mature just now, I understand music better, I feel it better, I understand the meaning of the composer and his language better. And so I consider myself a much better musician, as I get older."

Biologist Ernst Mayr admits to a lower level of performance and certain memory lapses. "There are many things where I am no longer as good as a younger person. The retrieval of names has become very much of a problem and some extremely well-known names are suddenly lost, I'm stumped and I can't think of them. I still have a very good memory for things from way, way back. Certainly things pop into my memory that happened to me in let's say, 1914. So there is still quite a bit of my storage, but it doesn't include names."

Oscar Shapiro has a similar problem. "After I finish a game I don't remember the whole game. Most chess players can play the game over immediately after they've finished it. And I can't do it. In some cases I don't even remember the name of the person I just played. And I've lost a great deal of memory for openings and that's very important. So, when I sit down to play, sometimes I have to improvise. I know more, but I think I execute less."

As these impressive elders are the first to admit, their old brains are not superior to young brains at everything. Their specialized knowledge built up over a lifetime in areas like music and chess—so-called crystallized abilities—makes them seem invincible. But when it's a question of processing new information quickly—using so called fluid abilities—it's a different story.

Psychologist Dr. Timothy A. Salthouse has been studying the cognitive differences between young and old at the Georgia Institute of Technology. He defines fluid abilities as "dealing successfully with novel situations, either artificial laboratory tasks, where the stimuli are familiar but the transformations that are required are novel, or you're dealing with totally novel stimuli in real-life situations. I think any time you're dealing with uncertainty on a continuous basis, the fluid abilities are very involved."

Crystallized abilities by contrast represent knowledge acquired over the years. Even something as mundane as knowledge of a one's neighborhood represents crystallized abilities. "In my case," says Salthouse by way of example, "I've lived in this area for many years now. I have a route that I follow to work. I don't have to think about it. I just get in the car and drive. I don't have to process information about whether to make a turn at a particular intersection. I can follow the over-learned route very automatically, almost without conscious processing.

"I know the names of most of my colleagues. It's something that is well over-learned. Much of what I teach is based on knowledge that I've acquired over the years, and so it's something that I don't have to think about a lot to have novel solutions to problems. So that's crystallized knowledge. Virtually everything that you do on a routine basis has become crystallized and set, so that you don't really have to engage in much processing in order to carry it out."

That's the sort of knowledge that stays with one throughout their life, a data bank from which information is constantly withdrawn and often replenished. "That type of knowledge," says Salthouse, "tends to either remain stable or increase in some circumstances. And we suspect it probably increases to a greater extent than we've been able to measure, because the knowledge is necessarily specific to a particular individual's interest and their specialization, and yet we don't have knowledge tests that represent that degree of detail right now. But it definitely holds up to a much greater extent than the fluid abilities."

Fluid abilities are more like quicksilver, slipping ever more quickly through the interstices of memory as we grow older. "Where we're talking about people of different ages measured at the same point in time," explains Salthouse, "there are very pronounced age-related declines in many fluid abilities. And I'm talking about things like reasoning, memory, the ability to spatially manipulate information so that you can see it from different perspectives or imagine a different orientation of an object."

So despite all the expertise we gain as specialists, we still lose our fluid abilities as we grow older. "Virtually everything that you do on a routine basis has become crystallized," says Salthouse. "As people develop specializations, they tend to concentrate in certain areas. So they can become experts in a given area, but they can still show normal age-related decline in other aspects of their abilities."

In a study of architects, Dr. Salthouse and his colleagues administered tests of spatial ability. The architects, who were presumed to have excellent spatial ability because of their profession, were asked to watch as a piece of paper was folded several times. Then, a hole was punched through the folded surfaces. The architects then had to decide what pattern of holes would result from that sequence of folds and hole punch.

In another test, they were asked to decide the correspondence between letters on a three-dimensional object and numbers on a flat surface. Both are tests of spatial ability the psychologists thought architects probably used in their normal professional lives.

"In that particular study," says Salthouse, "we found that the architects showed the same type of age-related decline in those abilities as unselected adults in our sample. Those were male college graduates who were comparable to the architects in background.

"The younger architects did better than the sixty-five-year-old architects. The middle-aged ones were in between. And the degree of age relationship was virtually the same as what we saw for non-architects. So that was a rather surprising finding."

Surprising or not, the age-linked decline in fluid ability has become a virtual paradigm. "Our general finding is that even people with a great deal of experience in a particular activity show age-related declines in some measures of performance that we think are related to that activity. For example, in the architect study, even architects would show some of the same kinds of age-related declines in tests of spatial ability that we think are relevant to the profession of architecture."

But all is not lost, for the skills and knowledge acquired over the years are used as a substitute for the facility of youth. "In terms of their professional work," says Salthouse, "I think that they are relying much more on crystallized intelligence, the knowledge base that they've acquired over the years. And that's much more important than the ability to perform these spatial ability tests, the fluid ability tests."

Young people unquestionably have an advantage when it comes to fluid abilities that involve carrying out novel tasks rapidly. Salthouse tests those abilities with tasks like the digit symbol test. Each of ten digits is paired in boxes with an arbitrary symbol immediately below it. Another set of boxes contain the digits, but not the symbols. The paired boxes in this case are empty. The test asks the subject to write the correct symbol for each digit as quickly as possible. Since the subjects don't know the pairs, they have to keep looking up to the set of boxes with the digits and the paired symbols.

"Whenever you're dealing with novel situations the fluid abilities are very involved," says Salthouse. "And it's an interesting test because it's something that is unfamiliar to people, the pairing of the digit and the symbol is arbitrary, so people haven't learned that in the past. And it requires people to be fast, but it also seems to involve working memory and you have to learn to associate these numbers with the digit symbol pairs."

Mehli Mehta's students may not have a fraction of his musical knowledge, but the digit symbol test cares nothing about that. In ninety seconds, the worst of Mehta's young students scored 55.... the best got 80. The maestro scored only 22. "And that's about what we would expect for someone of that age," says Salthouse. "The averages in our laboratory and in nationwide samples are usually around 60 or 70 for people in their twenties, and we found that the scores go down about one item every two or three years. Despite his genius in music, Mehta's brain is simply not working as fast as those of his students.

Salthouse has developed even more revealing tests of mental decline. In what can only be described as a fiendish computer test, subjects are asked to carry out several novel tasks at once. It's a challenge old people find quite hard. But young people find it relatively easy.

It's called synthetic work and requires the subjects to do four different actions at the same time. On the top left of a computer screen is a memory task. It consists of a set of letters. Immediately below is a probe letter. The letters disappear from the screen and the subject must decide whether the probe letter is in the set. If it is, then you push the button below labeled "yes." If it's not, you click on "no."

Immediately below the "yes, no" buttons is a visual monitoring task. A line moves to the left or the right and the subject must press reset before it reaches the end to push it back to the middle.

But that's only the beginning. Subjects have to simultaneously carry out some rather difficult arithmetic problems in yet another part of the screen, all the while listening for a high-pitched tone. If the tone is in fact high-pitched, then another button is to be pressed. All four of those activities are to be done at the same time.

It's a bit like juggling, riding a unicycle, playing a harmonica, and balancing your checkbook—all at the same time. Even the most accomplished seventy-year-olds have trouble doing two tasks, let alone four. Why do smart elderly people—even those completely familiar with computers—find this test difficult?

Dr. Salthouse offers this explanation: "We're taking all of the benefits of their lifetime accumulation of experience away from them, testing their powers, or at least we think we are testing their powers independent of any experience that they've acquired. It's a very stressful, demanding activity, and there are very large age differences. I think it has something to do with the fact that the older brain is just less efficient, and dealing with information it's slower in processing, it has problems maintaining some information while you're carrying out processing of other information. And there are very large age differences."

But for every problem there is usually more than one solution. Older people find ways to compensate for their slower brains.

"We're very interested in the area of accommodation, of compensation: how people can maintain a high level of functioning despite declines in certain aspect,." says Salthouse. "There are actually very few situations where we've been able to identify what the compensatory mechanisms are. One particular example in research of mine is in the area of typing, of transcription. There we found that young and old typists were able to type at the same speed, despite the older typists being much slower at being able to type a single key in response to a letter, or rapidly tap-tapping their finger. They were slower at things that are relevant to typing, but they were performing at the same overall speed in typing because they seemed to be looking farther ahead as they were typing.

So that's a compensatory-type mechanism. We think that there are similar things in many areas that people engage in."

Fortunately, for the most part, life doesn't demand we continually solve totally novel and fluid problems, certainly not four at a time. For much of life we can get by using our largely crystallized knowledge in certain areas—using words and numbers, reasoning, and navigating familiar spaces.

For researchers seeking understanding of the aging brain, a central question is how well do these everyday core skills hold up over time? Most of what is known has been learned from the people in the longest-running, continuous psychological experiment in history—the Seattle Longitudinal Study of Aging—begun in 1956.

Every seven years since, subjects have returned for a grueling test of their cognitive abilities. Researcher Warner Schaie hoped the study would solve the central mystery of the aging mind. "I started the study," explains Schaie, "because I observed that there were some old people who were still very bright and sharp and led exciting lives, while others were doddering old fools. And something had to happen to make that difference, and what that's really formed the basis of my life's work."

Schaie, who started this monumental project as a graduate student, has grown old doing it. Now in his seventies, he continues the study with his wife, Dr. Sherry Willis. The prevailing wisdom when Dr. Schaie started the project was that mental abilities would decline steadily from the twenties onwards. But the only way to know for sure was to follow individuals, lots of them, over their lifetimes. So Schaie set out to build a unique record of a person's intellectual performance, to see which areas declined and when.

The volunteers submitted to a full battery of cognitive tests. Everything from musty arithmetic skills originally learned in elementary and high school, to abilities used throughout life, like recognizing and expressing words. They also tested skills like spatial orientation.

"Spatial orientation is your ability to hold in mind an object and envision how it looks from different spatial orientations," says Willis. "This is what you do when you look at a road map and decide whether to turn left or right. This is what you do when you walk into a building and you see one of those 'you are here' signs that you're supposed to figure out where to go. It's a very important skill that we use in everyday life but most people aren't very conscious of it."

Another skill they tested was inductive reasoning—the ability to recognize patterns in our world. "Inductive reasoning is the ability to find rules and regularities," says Schaie. "You pick up a pattern, in other words. It's one of the most basic aspects of trying to solve any problem. For example, if you were to look at a bus schedule you might be able to recognize by scanning it, that there's a bus every hour. And now you no longer have to worry about looking up the precise bus because you know when it's going to be leaving."

Schaie expected these abilities would decline steadily with age from the twenties onwards. But as the data poured in, he began to realize this wasn't so. Remarkably, on most tests, whether they involved spatial relationships—the skill needed to get around—or the ability to pick up patterns in bus timetables, most people got more or less the same scores at age sixty as they had at twenty.

"In fact," says Schaie, "for most abilities, significant decline did not occur until the sixties or at least for some, like verbal meaning, until the seventies were reached. The other interesting finding was that for some of these, the peak of performance was not in the twenties but actually occurred in the thirties and forties, so that there was initially some gain. So the youngest groups, actually over the first period that we followed them, showed gain rather than decline."

Most people then were able to maintain their cognitive skills into their sixties, and those individuals who showed a marked decline, Schaie and Willis believe, probably had some pathological process operating. "It's simply not normal to show change on these basic intellectual skills until the sixties are reached," they say.

Past sixty, individual differences become very pronounced. "That period from the sixties to the eighties is where you get this tremendous variability. Once the eighties are reached, you find that virtually everybody has experienced some decline. And again, then you find that changes in the physiological infrastructure make it almost impossible to function at the level that was true in mid-life and early old age. But there are vast individual differences, because there are some people who clearly start declining in their sixties, while others really do not decline significantly until their early eighties are reached."

But again, there are many different patterns of decline. "It also depends to some extent on what kinds of abilities are supported and are practiced in your particular lifestyle," says Schaie. "So you may find that people decline in some abilities and maintain others, simply because they practice them. Now, some people have argued that what's going on here is a principle of selectivity and optimization, that people unconsciously realize that they cannot maintain all their skills, so they concentrate on some that are most critical to their particular lifestyles."

Preservation of some abilities also seems to be favored. "Certainly for verbal behavior you find that probably still about half the population has not shown any decline that could be reliably defined for an individual," continues Schaie. "On the other hand, by the eighties, virtually everybody has shown some decline on a skill such as inductive reasoning."

Gender differences also seem to play a role in the various patterns of decline. Men, for example, demonstrate stronger spatial orientation abilities than women until their sixties. "We found was that men, on average, are functioning at a higher level than women in young adulthood and middle age," says Willis. "And then when we reach mid-sixties, which is when spatial ability begins to decline, we see both genders declining, and the gender gap does not diminish or increase. It goes down in parallel. So the gender differences are maintained even as decline occurs. But they do not seem, at least through the sixties and early seventies, to either become bigger or smaller."

Gender differences also occur in a phenomenon known as terminal decline. "When we reach the seventies and certainly the eighties, then we have to become increasingly aware of what's called the gender differences in life expectancies, which are on average maybe seven years," says Willis. "And so men become increasingly closer to death, and therefore the phenomena that's sometimes called terminal decline can come into play, and that a number of years before a person actually dies, unless it's a death from a disease rather than an accident, there is some data that shows that people drop in certain abilities as they come closer to death."

Abilities across the board decline, but not everyone loses the same skills at the same time. "Individual differences become very pronounced," notes Schaie, "because it's really the period from the sixties to the eighties where you get this tremendous variability. Once the eighties are reached, you find that virtually everybody has experienced some decline. And again, then you find that changes in the physiological infrastructure make it almost impossible to function at the level that was true in mid-life and early old age. But there are vast individual differences, because there are some people who clearly start declining in their sixties, while others really don't decline significantly until their early eighties are reached."

By the eighties, virtually everyone had at least one area of significant loss. Schaie found in general that the people whose skills held up longest were well-educated, middle class, enjoyed good health, and, perhaps most interestingly, had a flexible approach to life. He measured flexibility with a special test which asked people to change all the upper case letters in a passage to lower case and vice versa. A task which most people find irritatingly difficult.

Flexibility, says Schaie, "is important because life is full of changes, and it makes a difference whether you are accepting of that and roll with the punches, or whether you fight it all the way. Some people have said that old age is not for sissies, and that's quite true. You have to accept the fact that the world is changing and that you need to do things differently. And those people who are fairly flexible, they actually may enjoy that. They may say, 'Gee, this is nice, it's interesting, it's new.' While somebody who is a very rigid personality style will say,

'Why do I have to go through this? Couldn't the world stand still and I get off?' And so in that sense we find that if a person gets more rigid as they get older, that actually is a poor indicator of maintenance of intellectual skills as well."

But if you're flexible, like eighty-nine-year-old Boston widow Mary Fasano, almost anything is possible. Fasano left school at fourteen to work in a cotton factory. After raising a family and working two jobs to put her children through college, she decided her turn had come.

"When I was seventy-one years old," she recalls, "my husband had passed away and that was when the idea came to me that it was my turn to go to school. And somehow or another I never thought of my age because I was always in good health. And it seemed as though I could do anything even at that age."

Fasano completed high school and then set her sights on a loftier goal: to earn her college degree from Harvard University. Day in day out, Fasano steadily gained credits towards her degree. "I worked hard at it, very hard, and as I got older, it became a little harder, and oh, it took a long time, it took me sixteen years."

At the age of eighty-nine, Mary Fasano became the oldest person ever to graduate from Harvard. And she's not finished yet. She's hoping to write her autobiography and she's taken up chess to keep challenging her mind.

Mary Fasano shows that the cognitive limits discovered by psychologists are no reason to give up. While an old person can't do everything as fast or do as many things at once as a young person, an old person can, if determined, go just as far.

Even the life choices we make, the partners we choose, can play a role in the way our skills decline with age.

"Interestingly enough," says Schaie, "it goes in the direction of the lower functioning partner at the beginning, then moving in the direction of the higher functioning one. So the smart thing to do is presumably to marry someone who's smarter than you are."

Genes also play a role. To determine just how great a role, as opposed to the impact of the environment, the National Institute of Aging funded a study of Swedish twins eighty years or older. It showed that individual differences in their cognitive abilities (how they acquire and use knowledge) depends as much on their genetic inheritance as on environmental factors. The study, by Gerald E. McClearn, Ph.D., of the Center for Developmental and Health Genetics at Pennsylvania State University, was the first to look at the influence of genes on many different aspects of cognition in older people. It confirmed patterns that have emerged from similar studies in younger and middle-aged people. Since cognitive function plays a crucial role in determining the quality of life for older people, understanding how cognition develops as people age could lead to beneficial interventions that might slow or reverse cognitive decline.

Dr. McClearn and his colleagues used as their database the Swedish Twin Registry, which has tracked 96 percent of all twins in Sweden. The study utilized 240 sets of these twins born before the start of World War I. They were an average age of eighty-three years old. To determine their cognitive abilities, twins were tested for verbal meaning, figure logic, block design, and picture memory. Analysis of combined scores of cognitive ability showed that their genetic inheritance accounted for 55 percent of the individual differences in ability, a result similar to that seen in middle-aged people.

The impact of the genetic inheritance on specific cognitive abilities, something that has not received a great deal of study in the past, was somewhat less than 50 percent but still highly significant. For both general and specific cognitive abilities, identical twins, as would be expected, showed much stronger similarities than did fraternal twins. Living together or sharing the same environment in later life did not account for any significant differences in the impact of the environment on cognition.

"In the group of Swedes that we studied," said Dr. McClearn, "even the effects of over eighty years of environmental influence didn't eliminate the impact of heredity on cognitive ability."

A wide range of environmental variables such as geography, education, socioeconomic status, nutritional habits, occupation, disease, and stress exposure might be expected to have substantial influences on cognition. Over the course of a lifetime, twins exposed to differing environments might be expected to display wide variances in cognition. Yet given the cumulative impact of a lifetime of environmental disparities, the study showed that the effects of environment on cognition are barely equal to the effects that genetic inheritance has on cognition.

Dr. McClearn and his colleagues' research is unique in that it looked in people age eighty and older at general intellectual ability and specific cognitive abilities such as spatial, verbal, and memory, and examined in detail each of the three separate areas of specific cognition. Previous twin studies had shown that general cognitive abilities are among the most inheritable behavior traits, with inheritable influence increasing from 20 percent at infancy to 60 percent in adulthood. This finding contradicted the commonly held assumption that environmental influence increases throughout the life span with a corresponding decrease in genetic influence. The study showed that the relative contributions of genetics and environment—about half and half—extends into very advanced age.

According to Dr. McClearn, "it is now becoming possible to identify specific genes which may be responsible for some of the differences in cognitive abilities. For example, certain forms of the ApoE gene have been associated with cognitive decline in older people, particularly in those with Alzheimer's disease."[45]

The results will lead to still more studies in hopes of learning more about the role of genetics and the aging brain. "The next step to better understanding genetic influences on cognition in older people is to conduct additional long-term studies on twins as well as studies using siblings and population-based samples," says Dr. Jared B. Jobe, Chief of the Adult Psychological Development Branch of the National Institute on Aging. "Discovering how we learn in old age could lead to a better understanding of how people can remain active and involved in society up to the very end of their lives."[46]

---

45. ApoE, Apolipoprotein E, is one of a family of proteins involved in the metabolism of lipids in human blood and body fluids. One variant of the gene known as e4 has been associated with increased risk for Alzheimer's disease.

46. "Even in Old Age, Genes Still Influence the Way We Learn, New Study Finds," *National Institute of Health Report,* June 1997.

7   Alzheimer's and the Chemistry of the Aging Brain

Studies of what successful older people can and cannot do have presented a challenge to neuroscientists studying the brain. What, they want to know, is going on in the brain to account for the patterns of declines? Why do crystallized abilities hold up and even improve with age, but fluid ones decline?

Changes in the aging brain have been detected that might account for the loss of mental speed. Dr. Marilyn Albert, a neuroscientist at the Harvard Medical School, has addressed the question of shrinkage in the brain. "The changes that we see are what we call atrophy, which is another way of saying shrinkage. And again it used to be thought that the whole brain was shrinking. Now we see that most of the changes are occurring in a part of the brain that we call the white matter."

Shrinkage can be easily seen in older brains. There are more fluid-filled spaces in the ventricles (openings) in the center and the regions at the top than in those of younger brains. There is less white matter, which is comprised of the forest of dendrites and axons that sprout from the neurons. Such shrinkage was believed to be one reason brains work less efficiently as they get older.

Another theory held that decline was caused by actual cell loss. Over time, a fair amount of neurons do die off. Until recently most scientists thought it was going on all over the brain from the moment of birth. That would be bad news, since the brain doesn't grow new neurons.

"Probably by the time you're five years old you've got virtually all of the neurons you're ever going to have," says Stanford University biologist Robert Sapolsky. "I mean people will debate just when the window closes, but pretty much early on you've got your entire bank account worth of neurons. What that means is if you lose a neuron, it can't be replaced."

This reality led neuroscientists to a depressing conclusion about neurons. "There was a general idea that you just lost them progressively over the life span," says Harvard's Albert. "And until very recently, that's what everybody believed and in fact most people don't even know that that concept has changed."

In the 1950s, brain researchers began working with a new tool called a microtome that enabled them to slice the brain into tissue paper thin slices. With it, scientists set out to try and measure just how many neurons were lost as people aged. Using the donated brains of deceased people aged nine to ninety, they sliced and diced, then mounted and stained the see-through, thin sections on slides. Then they counted what they saw under the microscope.

The results were shocking. In the elderly, it appeared that up to 40 percent of the neurons in the cortex, the outer layer, the thinking part of the brain, had been lost. Here was a compelling reason, some argued, to expect lower mental ability. But in the last decade, scientists have concluded these estimates were wrong.

The harvested brain cells were a broad spectrum mix from the brains of normally aging individuals and from patients who had died of Alzheimer's disease, which causes massive cell loss. But Alzheimer's is not the same as normal aging. And so researchers recently went back and repeated the cell counts, this time excluding people who had died with Alzheimer's. New imaging technology enabled them to get much more accurate estimates of surviving neurons. And it turns out we do not lose brains cells in droves as we get older.

A recent study confirmed the fact that increasing age does not mean increasing loss of tissue. Healthy eighty-five-year-olds don't lose brain tissue any faster than healthy sixty-five-year-olds, according to a study published in the December 1998 issue of *Neurology.* "People assume that we lose brain tissue faster as we get older, but this study shows that's not the case for those in good health," said neurologist Jeffrey Kaye, M.D., director of the Aging and Alzheimer's Center at Oregon Health Sciences University and the Portland Veterans Affairs Medical Center. Kaye and his colleagues initially tested healthy people ages sixty-five to ninety-five. Those showing signs of Alzheimer's disease or other dementia were excluded from the study because these disorders cause the brain to shrink. The study also excluded those with a history of diseases that might affect the brain, such as diabetes, hypertension, and stroke.

Researchers performed ongoing cognitive tests, and those who developed signs of dementia were also excluded from the study. The remaining forty-six participants were followed for an average of five years. Changes in brain volume over time were measured with magnetic resonance imaging (MRI) scans.

"The common perception that cell loss accelerates with age may be due to problems with previous studies," Kaye said. "Studies showing large differences in brain volumes in younger elderly people and the older elderly may have included many people who were destined to develop Alzheimer's disease. They may have already had significant losses in brain volume, even though no one would have detected yet that they had the disease."

For the healthy people in Kaye's study, the rate of brain tissue loss was small—1 percent or less per year. "This study implies that brain health continues well into the extremes of our current age span," Kaye said. "It suggests that we can age normally forever. On the other side of the coin, these people are still at risk of developing dementia."

Kaye also believes that understanding how the healthy brain ages also helps researchers understand how diseases affect the brain. "For example, if people have an accelerated rate of tissue loss in the brain, that may tell us they are going to develop dementia," he said. "This could help us identify people to participate in studies to determine whether new treatments are having an effect on the brain. Right now, claims that a drug is preventing the progression of the disease in the brain can't be substantiated."

The study measured changes in total brain volume. "More research is needed to determine whether the loss of volume is due to loss of neurons, the nerve cells that most people think of as 'brain cells,' or to loss of glial cells, the supporting tissue in the brain," Kaye said.[47]

"The latest thinking," says Marilyn Albert at Harvard, "is that in the cortex there's actually a minimal amount of neuronal loss. If you count a whole variety of brain regions you don't see much change in the cortex, which is the complicated part that has to do with elaborate thinking, as people get older. There are certain structures that are deep in the brain that are important for producing chemicals that go to the cortex that do have neuronal loss. But those structures are small and we think that maybe we can do something to alter those chemical changes. And that means that we might be able to develop ways of intervening, because if the nerve cells are there in the cortex to receive the chemical transmission, then we might be able to change the way that people alter their thinking as they get older."

The very fact that some regions of the brain lose nerve cells as we age and others do not represents an experiment of nature that researchers hope to use to the brain's advantage. It could, for example, account for the seemingly great variation in the way people's brains age. In one study Dr. Albert tested a mentally sharp, physically healthy group of oldsters. It was called the MacArthur study.

"We identified people who we defined as being successful agers," says Albert. "These were people who were doing well cognitively and physically. And then we followed them over time, and we looked to see what predicted who was

---

47. "Healthy Aging Brains Don't Shrink Faster," *American Academy of Neurology,* December 17, 1998.

going to continue to function successfully. And we found four things. One was higher levels of education. The second was higher levels of physical activity. The third was better lung function. And the fourth was something that we called self-efficacy, which was the feeling that what you did made a difference to what happened to you, sort of a feeling of control. And our hypothesis is that each of those things affects the brain in a slightly different way. And if each of those things together are operating, then you're much more likely to be cognitively well as you get older."

Albert believes that each of those four elements actually helps make beneficial changes to the brain. For the brain, researchers discovered, is highly adaptive.

"As you use your brain," explains Albert, "you're strengthening connections between nerve cells. And if you think that throughout your life you're exposed to insults of various kinds, and that threatens those connections, the more connections you have, then the more they are likely to be there after some slight insult."

Albert offers the effect of education on the brain. "Our hypothesis is that if you have higher levels of education, you are more mentally active throughout your life, so you do things that continue to stimulate the brain. You read. You talk with friends about interesting things. You use your brain actively. And that might actually mean that there are connections in the brain that are strengthened. And therefore, when you have some slight insult, the brain is much more likely to recover."

One of the most interesting studies to affirm this idea began in a convent in Mankato, Minnesota, in 1987. Here, Dr. David Snowden, an epidemiologist at the University of Minnesota, compared the disease and death rates of a more educated group of nuns against those with less education. All of the nuns belonged to an order called the School Sisters of Notre Dame. Some thirty-five hundred young women had joined the order in the early years of the twentieth century. Many went on to earn college degrees and to teach school, others became cooks, gardeners, and housekeepers for the order. Nearly one-third of the women were still alive in 1993, when the study was published. They ranged in age from 75 to 103.

The nuns provided an almost perfectly balanced mix of characteristics against which to match the effects of education on aging. Here was a group of women from similar backgrounds that had led remarkably similar lives since the age of twenty. Their meals had come from the same kitchens, they had shared the same living quarters, had access to the same health care.

The initial comparison indicated that a higher level of formal education appeared to be related to longevity with good mental and physical functioning. Snowden wondered about the reasons for the connection. In 1991, he joined a team of researchers at the Sanders-Brown Center on Aging at the University of Kentucky to pursue that question. Here the focus of the study shifted to the brain and the question of how the nuns' early lives might affect the cognition and function as they aged.

"We want to find out what causes Alzheimer's disease," says Snowden, now an associate professor of preventive medicine at the University of Kentucky. "In the long term we want to find out what promotes a long, healthy, high-functioning life."

The new study was dubbed the School Sisters of Notre

Dame Health and Aging Study. From the limited numbers in Mankato, the nun study has expanded to include hundreds of sisters in the Notre Dame convents of Milwaukee, St. Louis, Baltimore, Dallas, Chicago, and Wilton, Connecticut. More than half of the participants, 550, agreed not only to take part in the study, but to donate their brains after death.

The more highly educated sisters lived approximately four years longer, with a good level of mental and physical functioning, than those who had less than a bachelor's degree. At every age, from twenty to ninety-five, the nuns with less education had twice the mortality rate of the more highly educated.

"One explanation for this might be that higher cognitive function is due in part to higher-educated people having jobs—as well as recreational activities—that keep them mentally alive," says Snowden. "Another line of evidence is that people who have a rich vocabulary early in life end up having high mental function later in life."

Snowden and his colleagues examined the words used in autobiographies written by the nuns at age twenty-one, and their mental function sixty years later.

"We also looked at what the sisters were writing at age twenty one, then looked again a what they were writing twenty-five years later at age forty-six. Those sisters who improved their vocabulary between ages twenty-one and forty-six had better mental function at age eighty," reported Snowden.

The relationship between education and Alzheimer's, which seems to be supported by this and other studies, however, is less certain. "My suspicion is that education has nothing to do with the pathology of Alzheimer's," says Snowden.

"It isn't that lower-educated people have more plaques and tangles, rather it may be that more highly educated people have better connected brain cells."

Snowden cites an earlier study by Robert Katzman at the University of California, San Diego, that found the synapses of more highly educated people to be much denser. "If other parts of the brain are well connected, " says Snowden, "the healthy parts of the brain may have a better chance of taking over the functions of the parts of the brain damaged by Alzheimer's."[48]

Harvard's Marilyn Albert's studies of an elderly Boston population seem to agree. "Having more education means not only that you develop your brain when you're young, but that you use it more throughout your life, and that produces some sort of protective mechanism that helps keep the brain from developing Alzheimer's disease," she says.

Using new imaging technology, called functional MRI, Albert and other researchers can now watch the living brain as it receives and processes information. To study memory in the brain, Albert and her colleagues ask people to perform memory tasks. In one, they are shown different scenes. Some of the scenes are repeated, some are new. Another task calls for the subjects to look at drawings of simple geometric figures.

"We look at what happens in the brain when they're doing these different tasks," explains Albert. "And what that tells us is what's going on in the brain when the brain is trying to re-

---

48. "Studies Show Mental Activity Helps Ward Off Alzheimer's Disease," *Odyessy—The Magazine of University of Kentucky Research*, Summer/Fall 1994.

member something versus when it's just looking at some simple thing that doesn't mean very much. And then we try to figure out what parts of the brain are active, how they're active over time, how they interact with one another."

Not surprisingly the researchers noted that younger people remembered more of the scenes than the older people. What the researchers found most interesting was that if both the elderly and the young remembered the scenes very well, they were able to see heightened activity in a region of the brain that is involved in memory.

"The part of the brain that's critical for memory, which is the hippocampus and the regions around it, are active in both the young and the elderly people if they're healthy," says Albert. "They're active to a very great degree, to approximately the same degree [in both young and old brains] as far as we can tell."

Once it was believed that all of the brain's neuronal circuits were hard-wired, like the telephone system, with fixed circuits that could never be changed. But in fact we have learned that neurons are amazingly adaptable. "We now know that there are multiple levels where neurons adapt," says Dr. Carl Cotman, professor of psychobiology and neurology at the University of California, Irvine. "And they engage in these plasticity mechanisms short term, so that they can change the strength of the connections. In the long term they can actually regrow new synapses, reforming in place of the old ones by a thing called sprouting. When one dies next to it, the healthy cell actually replaces the circuit and rebuilds it back again. And then with minor interventions, it's actually been shown recently, including spinal cord, that you can regenerate the process. You can't necessarily bring the cell back if it's cut, but it'll actually grow back again with proper stimulation."

The brain also needs fuel to stay alive and function. Glucose is that fuel. "The brain totally depends on external glucose," explains Cotman. "If it doesn't have enough energy from glucose, it's in trouble. It also needs oxygen to make all of its proteins. They're all made in the cell body, and have to be transported all the way down the spinal cord. This is no small feat. Imagine a zebra, or a giraffe, or a whale—what a trip that is for a little protein to start off in the cell body and to go all the way down to the tail region. Then they've got to keep track of what's in all those processes so it acts as a total unit."

The entire system is extraordinarily complex. The brain, for example, is sealed off by the blood-brain barrier. This prevents the immune system that protects the body proper from attacking brain cells as foreign invaders. Breaks in the blood-brain barrier can send floods of scavenging antibodies into the brain where, mistaking them for disease agents, they will attack neurons.

Free radicals pose another threat to the neurons. The brain, in fact, faces a series of challenges that are immense. "And," points out Cotman, "if those challenges aren't met, any one of them will lead to a dysfunction."

In studying both normal and diseased brains, researchers have begun to understand the challenges every neuron faces. From the time we are born until we die neurons are fighting for survival. And they don't give up without a long and bitter struggle.

Part of that process can be seen under the microscope. Neurons exposed to toxic chemicals will start to retract their dendrites, which literally disappear. Eventually, the cell body itself comes under attack. At a certain stage a self-destruct program kicks in. But even then the neuron can take years to die.

"The neuron knows that it is in trouble," says Cotman. "So what it does is it has its own little garage and repair shop. And what's exciting to me about that is, it means that the neuron is struggling at that survival level, trying to stop it's degener-ation and trying to arrest the program that's causing it to de-generate.

"The neuron actually has everything in there to keep itself going, short of being blown out of the water. There's a whole series of stress activation pathways that start at the cell body, on the membrane. Give the membrane a signal that the cell's in trouble, and it will then start to generate a response back again to essentially start the program going. Then it checks at every single point in the program to make sure that it should go on to the next step. It's basically what we think is an apop-tosis decision cascade."

Apoptosis, Greek for "falling leaves," is the natural de-generation of a cell. It's literally a program that calls for the cell to commit suicide if it is beyond repair. Some re-searchers call it "programmed cell death." Cotman believes apoptosis is a prominent mechanism in the aging process. He also believes it to be a beneficial process because it eliminates the weak cells. If it gets out of control, then it's a disease.

Neuroscientists like Carl Cotman believe that the best chance of combating both Alzheimer's disease and the cog-nitive declines of normal aging may be in trying to help the neuron help itself. Neurons need just the right balance of chemicals to thrive and communicate with other neurons. Some of these chemicals they manufacture themselves, but others come from elsewhere in the body and from the foods we eat.

Even a brain without Alzheimer's disease has to face constant challenges as it ages. For we ask an enormous amount of our brains. "You can't do the fancy stuff your brain does without paying a price, and that bill comes more and more often as we age," says Stanford's Robert Sapolsky. "The brain has demands on it unlike any other organ in the body, as a result, it's got metabolic costs unlike anywhere else in the body, and metabolic costs wind up translating into vulnerability."

Sapolsky and other neurobiologists are trying to find the answers to a number of intriguing questions about the brain. "Why do we lose neurons when we age? And compared to other parts of the body, why do we lose more cells in the brain? Or why do they sustain more damage, more impairment of their function?"

The answer is surprisingly obvious. The neurons are called upon to do far more than any other cell in the body. "Basically because your brain does stuff your liver wouldn't dream of doing," says Sapolsky. "I mean, your liver wouldn't try calculus. Your liver wouldn't try coordinating all the muscles in your body. Your liver wouldn't try composing sonnets. It's a part of the body where you generate these things called oxygen radicals over the course of a lifetime. It's a part of the body where you slowly accumulate damage.

"You know, basically you will see something like cardiac arrest. Your heart stops beating. We all learn from "ER" and everywhere else: If you don't get the heart beating again in a couple of minutes, you start getting permanent damage. Where is the damage first? In your brain. Every single cell in your body is equally deprived of oxygen. It's a neuron that goes first because it's living in the fast lane. You can't do the fancy stuff your brain does without paying a price. And that bill comes more and more often as we age."

Stress, recurring in greater and lesser degrees over a lifetime, is thought to be another reason some brains might age faster than others. Stress can erase memory the way a blackboard can be wiped clean. Remember the nervousness and stress induced by school examinations. Thoroughly memorized answers to test questions flew out of your head, no matter how hard you chewed the pencil end. Then, twenty minutes after the exam ended, the elusive answers popped back into your memory—too late, of course, to help with your test score.

"We actually understand the biology now of why those neurons are not pulling out those memories," says Sapolsky. "In a longer-term sense, though, we are learning more about the ability of stress to accelerate aging of the brain, especially the part of the brain associated with memory. In that regard, stress is certainly bad for memory at the time of life where it's hardest to retrieve, in old age. We're certain of that in rodents. There's pretty good hints of that in primates. The first hints in humans are just beginning to come out."

Sapolsky does not believe that the ordinary stress of daily life, traffic jams, an abusive boss, or petty annoyances are going to accelerate aging in the brain. Nor is there any evidence that stress can cause Alzheimer's disease. Nevertheless, some people experiencing major levels of stress or otherwise generating large amounts of stress hormones may pay a price in the memory centers of the brain.

Researchers are particularly interested in that class of hormones secreted during stress. Steroid hormones called glucocorticoids can damage neurons in the parts of the brain that are very relevant to learning and memory. Originally seen in animal research, there is a growing belief that these kinds of neuronal damage may not be limited to laboratory rats but may affect the human brain as well.

Still, these hormones are essential for surviving acute stress, enabling animals, including humans, to fight or evade a predator or other threat. Called "the flight or fight" reaction, they mobilize energy, increase the readiness of muscles, and turn off nonessential body systems. In a short-term emergency, these hormones play a crucial adaptive function. But if they are elevated for too long, neurons can be damaged.

"It's looking as if this class of hormones secreted during stress can damage neurons in one part of the brain and in the part of the brain very relevant to learning and memory," says Sapolsky. "What seems to be the case is they cause a little bit of an energy shortage in neurons in this part of the brain. Nothing catastrophic, but they just constrain the neurons a bit in their ability to absorb and store energy. And what you get is a neuron, when it winds up having one of those tough days that neurons often do (because they do very fancy stuff that costs a lot), it takes them a little bit longer to clean up a class of neurotransmitters that could potentially be damaging. It takes them a little bit longer than usual to pump out some calcium ions that could potentially be bad news; a little bit longer to clean up oxygen radical damage. Every step is a little bit more costly, nothing fatal, except enough of this over enough time and a neuron drops off here and there. That seems to be the mechanism."

Even the events that promote neuronal health, often come with a negative flip side. One of the major challenges for brain researchers has been determining how fast it ages, and how the aging process differs among individuals. For years the answers were elusive. Now, according to Sapolsky, what most researchers had intuited is now pretty well supported by research. "Stimulation, novelty is great for an aging brain, great in terms of function, great in terms of neurons actually growing new processes, things of that sort. Great. Go get stimulated. That's wonderful.

"But what lots of us also know is, when there is too much stimulation we're not talking stimulation any more. We would now call that stress. Where is the dividing line? That's a real tough one. And basically, that's as tough for people looking at brain aging as for those looking at child development, where in both cases you need stimulation but not too much.

"Where is the dividing line? Nobody knows. Nobody knows in part because the research is very tough. Nobody knows, even more importantly, because we differ from one to another tremendously as to where it stops being stimulation and when it starts being bad news stress. Or at the other end, where it becomes under-stimulation, a paucity of input. It's real hard to tell. Get the right middle zone and the brain does wonderfully. Too much or too little, bad news."

Much of the current work in this area borders on the paradoxical, for virtually the only place to gain any sort of insight into the question of stimulation versus stress is from the developmental psychologists. Instead of looking at old geezers with aging brains, they look at the early years of life. They look to see how children develop what psychologists call a schema, a notion about how some facet of the world works. And if every time a child examines that part of the world, that schema, and the answer is the same (yes, this is how things work), the result is boredom. But give the kid what psychologists term a "moderately discrepant input," (things are just a little bit different), and the result is quite different.

"Kids smile," continues Sapolsky. "Their heart rate goes up, that sort of thing. Show them a face where one of the eyes is a little bit higher than the other, and this one-year-old can't get enough of it. 'Oh, I didn't know faces could be that way also.' Show them a new stimulus that's not a little bit discrepant but major-league discrepant. Show them some Picasso face with two eyes on one side, and they don't smile and get stimulated; they burst into tears. What you want is something that just pushed the envelope a little bit each time, from what they thought used to be the norm. That could count as new, wonderful music. This could be a new type of food to eat. That's a new way to think about a novel idea. Just a little bit different. But, a big discrepancy, a big discontinuity, that's when people start thinking of it as stressful."

While some chemicals like stress hormones can chip away at neurons, others protect and nourish them. One hormone that seems to be crucial to the health and survival of neurons is estrogen. Canadian researcher Barbara Sherwin of McGill University in Montreal became especially interested in estrogen's effects on the brain when she started hearing stories from women who no longer had the hormone. They had had their ovaries surgically removed, abruptly shutting off their brain's supply of estrogen.

"In interviewing them and working with them I was so impressed by the frequency with which they would come in and say, 'I've lost my memory, I just can't remember things anymore.'" Could it be true that eliminating estrogen can harm a woman's memory? Scientific evidence had already suggested that estrogen played an important role in memory, regulating chemicals that neurons use to communicate. Researchers have long known that the density of dendrites increases wildly when neurons are exposed to large amounts of estrogen. "So here you have a hormone that can actually affect the architecture of neurons in such a way that it increases the possibility that neurons are going to communicate with each other, so it enhances conversation between neurons which is really important for optimal brain functioning," notes Sherwin.

If estrogen has such a powerful positive effect on neurons, then it would make sense that the brain might notice its absence. After puberty, all human brains are exposed to estrogen. But while men continue to synthesize this vital chemical from testosterone all their lives, women are cut off once they reach menopause.

If losing estrogen really did impair memory, then half the population would potentially be affected to some degree. So Sherwin designed a groundbreaking experiment. She gave cognitive tests to women before gynecological surgery when their brains were still exposed to estrogen, and again afterwards when the supply was cut off following removal of the ovaries. A key mental skill declined.

"Those findings were very compelling," says Sherwin. "There were decreases on the tests of verbal memory that we gave them."

Since a drop in estrogen appeared to reduce mental skill,

Sherwin wondered if she could reverse the loss by replacing estrogen. So following surgery, she gave half the women estrogen. The other half received a placebo. The results were remarkable.

"The group that got estrogen," noted Sherwin, "their test scores were restored to pre-treatment levels, whereas the group that received the placebo, the decrement was maintained. That really did convince me that this was a real phenomenon."

Since some women going through normal menopause complain of cognitive losses, Sherwin's work has attracted a lot of interest. Never before had a hormone been shown to restore cognitive performance in healthy people. And researchers are investigating another possibility: that estrogen may turn out to protect women against Alzheimer's disease as well.

Alzheimer's is twice as common in women as men and the post-menopausal drop in estrogen may be part of the reason why. It is the most frightening of the dementias that attack the aging brain. Dementia is a broad catchall term for "a group of symptoms characterized by a decline in intellectual functioning severe enough to interfere with a person's normal daily activities and social relationships."[49]

Alzheimer's disease afflicts at least four million aging Americans. The actual number is unknown for Alzheimer's is not reported on death certificates. Surveys in various communities vary greatly. Some have reported the percentage of people eighty-five and older with any type of dementia in-

---

49. "Alzheimer's Disease, Unravelling the Mystery," *NIH Publication No. 95-3782*, October 1995.

cluding Alzheimer's to be in the 25 to 35 percent range. Others have been far higher. One Boston study of people eighty-five and older found the percentage with Alzheimer's alone to be 47.2 percent.[50]

The progressive, degenerative brain disorder now called Alzheimer's disease has been known since ancient times, its symptoms recorded by the Greeks and the Romans. In the sixteenth century, Shakespeare wrote of old age as "second childishness and mere oblivion," suggesting the symptoms of Alzheimer's were known in Elizabethan England. But it was not until the beginning of the twentieth century that the characteristic symptoms acquired their name, when a German physician, Alois Alzheimer, linked the symptoms to specific signs of damage in the brain. Dr. Alzheimer had a fifty-some-year-old patient who suffered from what appeared to be a form of mental illness. But when she died in 1896, an autopsy found dense deposits, now called neuritic plaques, outside and around the nerve cells in her brain. Inside, the cells were twisted strands of fiber called neurofibrillary tangles. These two physical markers, which are only revealed by autopsy, remain the only means of a definitive diagnosis of Alzheimer's disease.

The symptoms, however, present a sad even tragic picture of a life savaged by progressive, irreversible declines in memory performance of routine tasks, time and space orientation, language and communication skills, abstract thinking, and the ability to perform even simple mathematical calculations. Even more tragic are the personality changes and im-

---

50. "Alzheimer's Disease, Unravelling the Mystery."

pairment of judgement that are often also part of the ongoing destruction of the once vital and unique human being.

"With Alzheimer's people, there's no such thing as having a day which is like another day. Every day is separate . . . It's as if every day you have never seen anything before like what you're seeing right now," said Virginia history professor Cary Henderson who was diagnosed with Alzheimer's disease at the age of fifty-five.

Henderson recorded his feelings in a tape-recorded journal, while in the early stages of the disease. "You just feel that you are half a person, and you so often feel that you are stupid for not remembering things or for not knowing things. . . . Just the knowledge that I've goofed again or said something wrong or I feel like I did something wrong or that I didn't know what I was saying or I forgot—all of these things are just so doggone common."[51]

Alzheimer's usually begins in the sixties, in a small percentage of people, and becomes increasingly prevalent in each subsequent decade and may take twenty years to exact its ultimate horrific toll. Each year about 100,000 people die of Alzheimer's or related pneumonias. The neuritic plaques and neurofibrillary tangles that produce its symptoms begin deep in the brain in a region known as the entorhinal cortex. From there it moves to the hippocampus, a major assembly point for memory formation. It then spreads gradually to other sites within the brain, and eventually moves into the cerebral cortex, the thin outer layer where language and reason are formed. In the regions attacked by Alzheimer's, some

---

51. Henderson, Cary, "Musings," *The Caregiver: Newsletter of the Duke Family Support Program*, 12(2), 1994.

neurons die, while many more degenerate and the synapses that connect the nerve cells are broken.

As the hippocampal neurons degenerate, short-term memory diminishes. Usually the ability to perform routine tasks also falters. Cary Henderson describes the frustration he feels when he tries such simple tasks as opening a can of dog food. "The best I could do was to try to dig a hole, make a little perforation and see if I could extend the side of it—and it was something like a panic. I'm too clumsy because of the Alzheimer's....Right now the doggie seems to be in fairly good shape. I'm not too sure I am."[52]

Spreading outward, the disease attacks the neurons in the cerebral cortex, robbing the victim of language skills.

"Lately I've had trouble with words (practically having to play charades)," says Letty Tennis, a North Carolina woman who also kept a journal of her dark journey into Alzheimer's disease. As the disease progressed, she recorded her lapses in judgment and the emotional outbursts that punctuate her daily life. "We had a great time shopping, but I bought everything in sight. My poor dear husband didn't stop me very much unless it was too outrageous and then I'd get very angry. I bought a pair of boots—galoshes really...and I told George it's something I've always wanted so we bought them and when we got home I had no memory of buying them—they were awful and cost $40....I used to be the sensible one in the family."[53]

As the disease progresses, behavior becomes more bizarre. Its victims grow increasingly agitated, wander about

---

52. Henderson, "Musings."

53. Tennis, Letty, "Alzheimer's Diary: I Have What!" *The Caregiver: Newsletter of the Duke Family Support Program,* 12(6) 1992.

with no idea of where they are going or where they are. In the end stages, Alzheimer's wipes out the ability to recognize even close family members and the ability to communicate at all. All sense of self vanishes into the limbo of despair that is Alzheimer's tragic closing chapter. The victim becomes completely dependent upon others for care.

This condition can continue for years, until death comes from pneumonia or other diseases. From the time of diagnosis until the end, the disease may last for twenty years, although the average length is thought to be on the order of four to eight years.

A great deal of research is aimed at finding the causes of the disease, learning the risk factors and improving diagnosis and treatment. Underlying all efforts is research into the basic biology of the aging nervous system, which as we have seen is being undertaken all over the world.

"We used to think estrogens influenced only sexual behavior; now we know they also influence learning and memory," says Professor Victoria Liune, of Hunter College in New York.[54]

About twenty years ago, Liune, then a young researcher at Rockefeller University turned up one of the first hints that estrogen might play a role in brain chemistry. Liune and colleague Bruce McEwen gave estrogen to female rats whose ovaries had been removed. They then looked for changes in an area of the brain thought to control reproduction. What they found, among other things, was an increase in levels of an enzyme known as choline acetyltransferase, a precursor

---

54. "Estrogen: A New Weapon Against Alzheimer's?," *Science*, May 2, 1997.

of acetylcholine, the biochemical messenger used to communicate nerve impulses between neurons.

It was an interesting discovery, but hardly groundbreaking. Some ten years later in the mid-1980s, Liune found laboratory evidence that estrogen protects neurons from the destruction that usually accompanies Alzheimer's disease. Dr. Howard Fillit, a colleague at Rockefeller, then designed a pilot program to study of the effect of estrogen on six elderly women suffering from Alzheimer's disease. One had been quiet, apathetic, and unable to learn pairs of words. After the estrogen treatment, she became much more alert, talkative, and able to remember the words after just a few trials. Fillit treated six other women and two of them showed an increase in their cognitive skills.

Buoyed by his findings, Fillit applied to several agencies for a grant to further study estrogen and Alzheimer's disease. He was turned down by everyone, including the National Institutes of Health. He was told, he recalls, his applications "had no scientific merit."

But several other small treatment studies have replicated Fillit's results and other studies offer hope that the hormone might prevent or delay the onset of Alzheimer's in women. In fact, there is growing interest in the use of estrogen in this area and a great deal of work has demonstrated a definite beneficial effect on the neurons and learning.

Among the most important of the recent studies was the National Institute on Aging's Baltimore Longitudinal Study on Aging. For forty years this program has observed many aspects of aging in over 2000 people. For sixteen years 472 women of that group were given estrogen replacement therapy and were found to have a more than 50 percent reduction in the risk of developing Alzheimer's. The women were examined in intensive two-and-a-half-day visits every two years, submitting to a battery of physical and cognitive tests to determine any onset of dementia.

"This finding gives us additional evidence that estrogen may play a role in warding off the onset of this devastating disease," said Dr. Claudia Kawas, one of the doctors conducting the study.

"Estrogen is a substance worthy of further study as a protective drug against Alzheimer's disease," adds Dr. John Metter, another member of the team, "because it has been shown to exhibit both antioxidant and anti-inflammatory activity, lower ApoE levels in plasma (certain forms of the ApoE gene have been linked to an increased risk of Alzheimer's in some people), as well as to enhance the growth of certain neurons that release a crucial brain transmitter known as acetylcholine."

And, concludes Dr. Kawas, "Estrogen has been shown to have a direct effect on brain structure and function, particularly for women. 'Designer' estrogen, drugs that are currently being developed by a number of pharmaceutical companies, could minimize estrogen's feminizing and other unwanted side effects and provide a potent strategy for both men and women in delaying or reducing death due to Alzheimer's disease in a large segment of the aging population. If these drugs can be synthesized, only with double-blinded clinical trials will we really know if these substances will be effective in the fight against Alzheimer's disease."[55]

---

55. "16-Year Study Is Further Evidence That Estrogen Replacement May Be Protective Against Alzheimer's Disease," NIA Report, June 1997.

What other naturally occurring chemicals might protect and nurture neurons? Carl Cotman is interested in a strongly protective chemical that the brain itself produces called Brain Derived Growth Factor. Growth factor can prevent dendrites from retreating and even help them grow back. Since neurons already made this chemical in small amounts, Cotman wondered if they could be encouraged to make more. Research in rats had already shown that exercise increased the blood supply to the rats' brain. Could exercise alone, Cotman wondered, increase production of this protective growth factor as well?

"We sort of suspected that there was a real benefit of exercise on the brain, and not just on the body and the muscle structure. And so we wondered what's this class of molecules that's really the best known things that a neuron can make? And it turns out; it's these growth factors. You infuse a growth factor into the brain and it saves dying cells, it stimulates growth, it stimulates regeneration. And so the idea was, maybe, just maybe, the brain is actually capable of regulating growth factors, through just being used, i.e., exercising. Just like a muscle gets stronger, maybe the brain can actually get stronger from exercise and keep its cells healthier."

In tissue culture, several growth factors protected the neurons from a series of insults from toxins. The cells also demonstrated a much higher survival level from free radical damage. Among the most effective was Brain-Derived Neurotrophic Factor, or BDNF. Cotman then designed a series of experiments to see if exercise did in fact cause the brain to increase levels of BDNF. It did, but the biggest surprise was that the increase was not just in the motor areas, it also increased it in areas involved in cognition and reasoning, in thinking and learning.

"And so that gets really exciting," says Cotman, "because just plain old activity is actually doing something to keep the health of the cognitive areas of the brain up and active and in better health."

If exercise affected the cognitive areas of rats' brains, what about humans? Cotman recruited eight hundred people from a large retirement complex. As is typical in most scientific experiments, the group was split in two. Half exercised on a daily basis. The other half, a matched group of otherwise healthy people of the same age, did not. Both groups were then given a battery of cognitive tests.

"We had some real exciting findings come out of that study," recalls Cotman. "The people that were in the exercise groups were cognitively better performers than the ones that weren't in there. So exercise by itself is associated with improved and higher performance cognition."

Cotman was suggesting that exercise didn't just increase the brain's blood supply. It also increased the amount of the brain's own chemicals that protect and repair neurons leading over time to improved cognitive abilities.

The findings, according to Cotman, are perfectly consistent with those found in animal studies. "BDNF, for example, is known to enhance learning. It's known to be essential for learning mechanisms in animals. So it's a nice thread from the beginning principle to the basic science level, up through humans. And that's what we're really trying to do in research, to make discoveries, figure out what they might mean, and then translate them finally to the human situation.

If confirmed, the implications are significant. And scientists like Cotman are already taking the results to heart. "I started becoming more of an adherent to exercise after what I found in our own data. You know if you find it you've got to believe in it. And so I exercise regularly. I also take antioxidants and a few of the other things that seem to have come out of the science."

Harvard's Marilyn Albert also is a convert. "Since we got our data I exercise everyday. I'm mentally active so I take care of that, but I do think that feeling differently about stress is important and I try to put that into action."

Aging researchers seem in no doubt. What some elders had already discovered by themselves has now been given scientific authority. The way to age well is through a life of intellectual challenge, healthy living, plenty of exercise.

And, of course, avoiding too much stress.

Despite the many studies and observations such as those just listed, it remains difficult to codify successful aging.

"One of the interesting things in this field is older people who have what's termed a sense of self-efficacy tend to do better," says Robert Sapolsky. "They are 'aging successfully.' That's the jargon that's popular these days. What's the self-efficacy business about? First pass at this was one straight out of classical psychology, an internal locus of control. You're the master of your fate. That sort of thing. That's a predictor of folks who do better."

But like so many assumptions in the field of aging, everything is not quite what it seems.

"There's a problem with that," notes Sapolsky, "which is aging is a time of life where there's lots of stuff, often with some pretty rough edges to it, that you in fact have no control over. And the last thing you want to do is counsel somebody to try to feel as if they should be able to control the uncontrollable. That's a prescription for disaster.

"What the more subtle studies show is the folks who are really doing well in terms of successful aging have the most accurate perception of their sense of control, the best fit between the reality and how they perceive it. They are not trying to control the impossible stuff. They are accommodating to the inevitabilities of aging. But the realms in which there's still something they can do, they go at it with a fighting spirit; they go at it with a proactive, optimistic style. That's the prescription for folks who are going to be doing terrifically in old age."

8 *Tomorrow*

As we enter the new millennium we are also crossing a watershed in human history. For the first time the likelihood exists that a child born in America today will live to see his one-hundredth birthday. There is also a better than even chance that at least one of his or her parents will achieve the Biblical three score and ten, and perhaps four million of that group will become centenarians.

Many social policy analysts consider the coming explosion of the elderly in America the equivalent of a new tidal wave of immigrants, with the power to forever change the social and cultural landscape. Consider that each day three thousand people turn sixty-five, and only two thousand over that age die. The net is a thousand new members of the elderly generation. In the next twenty years the sixty-five-plus population in America will grow by 71 percent, more than twice the growth rate of the general population. By the year 2020, one out of every six Americans will be over sixty-five.

Genetics will play a large role in determining just who will enter that select group. After all, if grandma lived to a ripe old age, so might you. That at least has been the prevailing wisdom. But in point of fact, lifestyle and location may play an even greater role than genealogy in determining longevity. A recent study in *The New England Journal of Medicine* states flat out that the United States may be the healthiest place on earth for old people. The report found that Americans who reach age eighty could expect to live about a year longer than the elderly in four other industrialized countries. The results were totally unexpected, since the United States trails many other countries in life expectancy measured from birth.

But those Americans who do make it to old age, do as well as or better than elderly people anywhere. "It's a surprise to us, and I think it will be a big surprise to the Europeans, who always argued that they are doing so much better than the U.S.," says Dr. Richard M. Suzman, head of the Office of the Demography of Aging at the National Institute on Aging.

One probable explanation for older Americans' longevity is the quality and availability of their health care.

"When people turn sixty-five, we become a country with universal health care," notes Kenneth G. Manton of Duke University, the study's principal author. "Other countries have it from birth, but they cap expenses, and that translates into delays."

Americans on Medicare get virtually any care they need— new knees, coronary bypass surgery, transplants, whatever—without long waits. Other countries hold down costs by limiting the availability of expensive services and requiring patients to queue up, sometimes for many months.

"Older people can tolerate waits less well," Manton said. "Being incapacitated while waiting for joint replacement surgery can have a disastrous effect on someone who is eighty."

Manton and fellow demographer James W. Vaupel of Odense University in Denmark looked at death records of people born between 1880 and 1894 in the United States, Sweden, France, England, and Japan. The data offers the first reliable comparisons between countries.

The study found that American women who turned eighty in 1987 were expected to live 9.1 more years, while men were expected to live 7 more years. Life expectancies for eighty-year-old women and men in Japan were 8.5 and 6.9 more years, respectively; France, 8.6 and 6.7; Sweden, 8.3 and 6.5; and England, 8.1 and 6.2.

The researchers also calculated the odds of surviving five more years at ages eighty, eighty-five, ninety, and ninety-five. Americans consistently did best. For instance, an eighty-five-year-old American woman has a 58 percent chance of living five more years, compared with 53 percent in France, 52 percent in Japan, 51 percent in England and 50 percent in Sweden.

When life expectancy is measured from birth, the United States trails Japan, France and Sweden and is locked in a virtual tie with England. Japanese women have the world's highest life expectancy at 83. An American woman's life expectancy is 79.8.[56]

---

56. Manton, Kenneth G., Ph.D., and Vaupel, James W., Ph.D., "Survival after the Age of 80 in the United States, Sweden, France, England, and Japan," *New England Journal of Medicine,* November 2, 1995.

The other major factor is that a generation that has devoted itself to eating right and keeping fit has a far better
chance of becoming centenarians than those who by circumstance or decision eat poorly and get little or no exercise. Thus, longevity may well be determined as much by
our own desires as by our genealogy.

Given the fact that we are all inevitably going to age, the
question becomes less one of quantity than of quality. How
good will life be for those of us who hit the century mark and
beyond? Will we roller-blade along on our replacement hips
and knees, our bones and muscles strengthened by hormone
and vitamin cocktails, our minds and memories enlivened by
Urdu lessons and games of virtual three-dimensional chess?

The idea is appealing, but still, 100 or 120 years is a long
time to live. Even setting aside the enormous social and
economic problems facing a nation with one-third of its citizens on social security and Medicare, will those who successfully meet the physical challenges of old age enjoy
their longer lives?

Getting older usually signifies more aches, pains, memory
problems, and other age-related discomforts. And these problems will not go away despite our lengthening life spans. But
that does not necessarily signify a decline in the ability to enjoy
life. Individual happiness according to a study reported in the
Journal of Personality and Social Psychology found that as
people get older, they become happier, not sadder. Psychologist Daniel K. Mroczek, Ph.D., of Fordham University, and Ful-
bright Scholar Christian M. Kolarz, B.S., of the University of
Warsaw in Poland examined the responses of 2,727 men and
women age twenty-five to seventy-four years old to a survey
to find out how much a person's age, gender, marital status,

education, stress, health, and personality (levels of extroversion, introversion, and neuroticism) affected their well-being.

"The older the person was, the more he or she reported positive emotions like cheerfulness, life satisfaction, and overall happiness within the past thirty days," wrote Mroczek and Kolarz. "And surprisingly, the younger participants reported more negative emotions, like feeling sad, nervous, hopeless, or worthless. We found that age still had an affect even when the other factors (gender, marital status, education, stress, health, or personality) were taken into account as possible influences."

Another surprise turned up among older men, especially the married ones, who reported being the happiest and having the least amount of negative emotions. Older women also reported more positive emotions than their younger counterparts. But age played no role among the women in their reporting of negative emotions.

"Those that were measured as the happiest were not only older and male, but were also married and more extroverted," said Dr. Mroczek. "We have seen this before in other research on age and well-being which found that relationships played a major role in determining the extent to which people gain greater regulation over their emotions as they age. It is possible that men are able to learn how to minimize negative emotions in their marriages.

"From our research," said the authors, "we have seen that older adults regulate their emotions more effectively than younger or middle-aged adults. We can propose that older individuals seem to be able to know, through their years of experience, what kinds of external events increase or decrease their positive and negative emotions. Therefore, they achieve a better 'emotional balance' by selecting people and situations that will minimize negative and maximize positive emotions."[57]

Amidst the flurry of studies and testing the elderly have been subjected to over the last decade or so, one single characteristic seems to typify those who are successful agers. Mental toughness is the trait shared by virtually all centenarians. "Strong personalities distinguish centenarians," says Leonard Poon, director of the Centenarian Project at the University of Georgia, the longest ongoing study of people one hundred and older in the nation. "They tend to be domineering. They tend to be what we call suspicious. Essentially they would not easily believe what you say. They want to verify what you say."

A deep and abiding spiritual belief is another distinguishing characteristic. "Religiosity was found to be an important factor in the lives of all centenarians," notes Poon. These older adults, regardless of whether they are black or white, are all very religious and it serves as a support system. We found this related to mental health. We did not find much depression among our centenarians."

The future, like the past, will be pretty much what we make it. But never before have we had the awesome, almost God-like ability to virtually double the human life span. For the first time in history control of the aging process lies in our own hands. Everything from complicated genetic technology to simple exercise, constant intellectual challenge, and a good diet can mean longer, healthier years. The only remaining question is how many of us will take advantage of the miracle that is being offered. For it will happen, and sooner rather than later.

---

57 *Journal of Personality and Social Psychology*, November 1998.

Selected Bibliography

Adler, Lynn. *Centenarians: The Bonus Years*. Health Press: 1995.

Amery, Jean. *On Aging: Revolt & Resignation*. Indiana University Press: 1994.

Austad, Steven N. *Why We Age*. John Wiley & Sons: 1997.

Bernstein, Carol and Bernstein, Harris. *Aging, Sex, & DNA Repair*. Academic Press, Incorporated: 1991.

Cavanaugh, John C. *Adult Development & Aging*. Brooks/Cole Publishing Company: 1992.

Chopra, Deepak, M.D. *Growing Old*. Harmony Books: 1993.

Cox, Harold G. *Later Life: The Realities of Aging*. Prentice Hall: 1995.

Cranton, Elmer and Fryer, William. *Resetting the Clock: 5 Anti-Aging Hormones That Are Revolutionizing the Quality & Length of Life*. M. Evans & Company Incorporated: 1996.

Driskill, J. Lawrence. *Adventures in Senior Living: Learning How to Make Retirement Meaningful & Enjoyable*. Haworth Press: 1997.

Ebersole, Priscilla. *Toward Healthy Aging*. Mosby-Year Book, Incorporated: 1997.

Elias, Jeffrey W. and Marshall, Philip H., Editors. *Cardiovascular Disease, Aging & Behavior*. Hemisphere Publishing Corporation: 1999.

Evans, William, Ph.D. and Rosenberg, Irwin H., M.D. *Biomarkers—The 10 Determinants of Aging You Can Control*. Simon & Shuster: 1991.

Finch, Caleb E. and Johnson, Thomas E., Editors. *Molecular Biology of Aging*. John Wiley & Sons: 1990.

Fossel, Michael, Ph.D., M.D. *Reversing Human Aging*. William Morrow: 1994.

Hayflick, Leonard, Ph.D. *How and Why We Age*. Ballantine Books: 1996.

Kanungo, M.S. *Genes & Aging*. Cambridge University Press: 1994.

Martin, George R.; Holbrook, Nikki J.; and Lockshin, Richard A., Editors. *Cellular Aging & Cell Death*. John Wiley & Sons: 1995.

McGuire, Francis A.; Boyd, Rosangela K.; and Tedrock, Raymond T. *Leisure & Aging: Ulyssean Living in Later Life*. Sagamore Press: 1999.

Medina, John J. *The Clock of Ages*. Cambridge University Press: 1996.

Moody, Harry R. *Abundance of Life: Human Development Policies for an Aging Society*. Columbia University Press: 1988.

Murphy, Donald J. *Honest Medicine: Shattering the Myths about Aging & Health Care*. Grove/Atlantic, Incorporated: 1996.

Naranjo, Claudio. *Melatonin & Aging Sourcebook*. Hohm Press: 1997.

Orlock, Carol. *End of Aging: How Medical Science Is Changing Our Concept of Old Age*. Carol Publishing Group: 1995.

Pipher, Mary. *Another Country: Navigating the Emotional Terrain of Our Elders*. Putnam Publishing Group: 1999.

Posner, Richard A. *Aging & Old Age*. University of Chicago Press: 1996.

Ricklefs, Robert E. and Finch, Caleb E. (Contributor). *Aging : A Natural History* (Scientific Amercan Library). W.H. Freeman: 1995.

Robertson, Joel with Monte, Tom. *Peak Performance Living*. Harper Collins: 1996.

Rowe, John Wallis and Kahn, Robert Louis. *Successful Aging*. Delacorte Press: 1999.

Rybash, John M. *Adult Development & Aging*. Brown & Benchmark: 1994.

Salthouse, Timothy A. *Adult Cognition: An Experimental Psychology of Human Aging*. Springer-Verlag New York, Incorporated: 1982.

Schulz, Richard and Salthouse, Timothy A. *Adult Development and Aging: Myths and Emerging Realities*. Prentice Hall College Division: 1999.

Schulz-Aellen, Marie-Francoise. *Aging & Human Longevity*. Birkhauser Boston: 1996.

Spence, Alexander P. *Biology of Human Aging*. Prentice Hall: 1994.

Suzman, Richard M.; Willis, David P.; and Manton, Kenneth G. (Editors). *The Oldest Old*. Oxford University Press: 1995.

Walford, Roy L., M.D. *Maximum Life Span*. W.W. Norton: 1983.

 *Index*

A

Actinomyces bacterium, 72
adeno-associated virus
    (AAV), 140-41
adenosine triphosphate
    (ATP), 124
Advanced Glyosylation End
    products (AGEs), 117
Albert, Marilyn, 197, 198,
    201-2, 205-6, 224
Alberts, Bruce, 89
Alternative Medicine, 145-46
Alzheimer, Alois, 216
Alzheimer's disease, 29,
    130-31, 196, 197-99, 200,
    209
    Brain-Derived Neu-
        rotrophic Factor
        (BDNF) experiments,
        222-24

brain shrinkage generally,
    197-201
education and, 202-5
estrogen, effects of, 220-
    21
nun population study,
    202-5
process, symptoms and
    effects of, 215-19
American Youth Symphony,
    168, 179-80
amyotrophic lateral sclero-
    sis (ALS), 126-28
Andersen, Ross, 142
apes, 38-39, 40-41, 42, 109-
    14
apoptosis, 208
architects, 184-85
Atomic Energy Commission
    (AEC), 52

Austad, Steven, 15, 37, 59-65

B

baby-boomers, 10
Bacillus sphaericus, 71-73
Baltimore Longitudinal
 Study on Aging, 220-21
Baltimore Sun, The, 49
Barrett-Conner, Elizabeth,
 150-51
bees, 56-57, 71-73
Bell, Graham, 74-75
Biosphere 2, 104-7
birds, 56
Bismarck, Otto, 174
Blackburn, Elizabeth, 162
Blackman, Marc, 146
Blumberg, Jeffrey, 129-30,
 133
Boley, Helen, 98, 100-101
Botstein, David, 87
brains, 15-16, 167-68
 Alzheimer's disease. *See*
  Alzheimer's disease
 apoptosis, 208
 Brain Derived Growth
  Factors, 222-24
 cell loss question, 171-72
 compensation in elders,
  187-88
 crystallized vs. fluid abili-
  ties, 182-87
 Diamond and Scheibel,
  work of, 168-75
 digit symbol test, 185-86
 education, effects of, 201-5

 exercise and neuron
  health, 222-24
 flexibility, 192-93
 gender differences, 191
 genetic factors, 194-96
 inductive reasoning, 189
 language learning, 171
 MacArthur study, 201-2
 memory study, 205-6
 mental decline, patterns
  of, 188-93
 neuron adaptability and
  health, 206-9
 old rats and new tricks,
  175-78
 reticular formation, 175
 retirement and work, 173-
  75
 shrinkage of, 197-201. *See
  also* Alzheimer's dis-
  ease
 spatial orientation, 184-85,
  189, 191
 stimulation and aging,
  172-75
 stress, effects of, 210-13,
  224
 Swedish twins, 194-96
 synapses, numbers of,
  170-71
 synthetic work test, 186-87
Bramlett, Martha, 24
breast cancer, 143
Brewer, Brian, 98
bristle cone pines, 57

British genealogical records, 44-45

Brown, James, 50-51

Brown University, 76-77

Brzezinski, Amnon, 153

Burns, George, 168

C

Caenorhabditis elegans worm, 86-95

Calment, Jeanne, 25-26, 33

Caloric Restriction diet (CR-diet)
  Biosphere 2 humans, 104-7
  monkey research, 109-14
  rat and mice research, 103-4, 107-9

Campisi, Judith, 13, 158-61, 164

cancer, 32, 130, 143, 155, 164-65
  tumor suppression and aging, 159

Cano, Raul, 71-73

castrated men, 155-56

cataracts, 31, 130

cats, 49-50

Cech, Thomas, 163

cell division and senescence, 157-60
  fibroblasts, 160-61
  Hayflick limit, 161, 162, 163, 164, 166
  telomeres and telomerase, 161-66

tumor suppression, 159

centenarians. *See* one-hundred-year-olds

Cerami, Anthony, 114-19

childbearing. *See* reproduction and childbearing

chimpanzees, 38-39, 40, 42, 47, 66

cholesterol, 98-101, 105

choline acetyltransferase, 219-20

Choy-Pik Chiu, 165

Clarke, Steven, 58

Cockburn, Alexander, 68

cognitive abilities. *See* brains

collagen, 63-65

compression of morbidity, 28-29

Cooper Institute of Aerobics Research (Dallas), 141-42

Cotman, Carl, 206-8

Cranton, Elmer, 145-46, 222-24

D

dehydroepiandrosterone (DHEA), 149-51, 154

diabetes, 112, 114-15, 118

Diamond, Jared, 37-39, 40-41, 42-44

Diamond, Marian, 168-75, 178

diet and nutrition, 15, 16
  Caloric Restriction diet

(CR-diet), 103-14
cholesterol, 98-101
folic acid, 131-33
glucose metabolism, altering of, 95-96
vegetables and fruit, 128-29, 133
vitamin B6, 131-33
vitamins C and E, 129-31
wine, 128-29
digit symbol test, 185-86
"disposable soma" theory, 35
Drosophila melanogaster flies, 78-83
Duke University Center for Demographic Studies, 29-30
Dunn, Andrea, 142

E
Einstein, Albert, 167
elephants, 47, 49, 56
eleven-year-olds, 21
Elliot, Mary Sims, 25
emotional state of elders, 230-32
Enquist, Brian, 50-51
Eos, 108
estrogen, 153
  brain, effects on, 213-15, 219-21
Ettinger, Bruce, 153
eunuchs, 155-56
Euplotes aediculatus, 163
exercise, 16-17, 31, 135-36,

143-44
brain neuron health, 222-24
hormone therapies doing the work of. *See* hormones
reversal of muscle loss, 137-39
vigorous vs. moderate, 141-42
women, strength training for, 136-39

F
Fasano, Mary, 193
fibroblast senescence, 160-61
fight or flight reaction, 69
Fillit, Howard, 220
Finch, Caleb, 21, 33, 56-57, 69-70
Finkelstein, David, 95
Fleming, James, 86
folic acid, 131-33
Frackelton, James, 145-46
free radicals, 16, 100, 107-8, 122-26, 207
  exercise and, 143
  Lou Gehrig's disease and, 127-28
French paradox, 128-29
Frost, Robert, 167
fruit flies, 14, 16, 78-83, 86, 92, 123, 125-26
fruits, 129, 133

G

Galloway, Alison, 42
genetic factors, 31-32, 34-36, 85, 228
  clock genes, 93-94
  cognitive abilities, 194-96
  fertility and longevity in women, 44-46
  fruit fly experiments, 78-83, 86, 92
  Human Genome Project, 84-85
  knockout technique in research, 76
  Longevity Assurance Gene (LAG-1), 75-76
  Lou Gehrig's disease, 126-28
  muscle and strength enhancement, 139-41
  nematode studies, 86-95
  p21 gene in humans, 76
  reproductive stress, 66-70
  Sapelo Island opossums, 61-65
  single-celled organisms, 73-75, 77-78
  SOD gene, 86
  telomerase gene therapy, 162-66
  Werner's Syndrome, 96-98
  yeast research, 75, 77-78, 87, 88, 162
Georgia Centenarian Study, 24-25, 232

Geron Corp., 163, 165-66
Gibbons, Whitfield, 51-56
Glenn, John, 143
glucocorticoids, 69-70
glucose metabolism, 95-96, 111-12, 114-49
Gompertz Mortality Model, 33
gorillas, 38-39, 40-41, 42, 66
Goubert, Pierre, 27
Grandma Moses, 167
grandmothers, 42-44
Greenough, William T., 16-17, 175-78
Greider, Carol, 162
guinea pigs, 48-49

H

Hamilton, James, 155-56
Harlem Jazz Legends, 168
Harley, Calvin, 166
Harmon, Mitchell, 146, 148
Harris, William, 98, 101
Hawkes, Kristen, 42
Hayflick, Leonard, 51, 66, 157-58, 161, 162, 163, 164, 166
health-care costs, 10, 228-29
Health Care Financing Administration, 10
heart disease
  cholesterol, 98-101, 105, 132
  folic acid and vitamin B6, 131-33
  homocysteine, 132

Hebrew Home for the Aged
(Boston), 22
Hekimi, Siegfried, 93-94
helicase, 97
Henderson, Cary, 217, 218
high density lipoproteins
(HDLs), 98-101
homocysteine, 132
honeybees, 56-57
hormones, 144-45
brain (cognitive) effects,
210-15, 219-21
dehydroepiandrosterone
(DHEA), 149-51
estrogen, 153, 213-15, 219-
21
human growth hormone
(HGH), 145-49
melatonin, 151-53
stress hormones, 210-13
testosterone, 153-56
horses, 47, 48-49, 80
houseflies, 119-21
How and Why We Age
(Hayflick), 51, 157-58
Human Genome Project, 84
human growth hormone
(HGH), 145-49
hydroxyl radical, 125

I
insulin-like growth factor
(IGF-1), 140-41

J
Jazwinski, Michal, 75, 77-78

Jobe, Jared B., 196
Johnson, Thomas, 14, 21, 85,
87, 90-93
*Journal of Obstetrics and
Gynecology,* 153
*Journal of Personality and
Social Psychology,* 230
*Journal of the American
Medical Association,*
131-32, 141

K
Katzman, Robert, 205
Kawas, Claudia, 221
Kaye, Jeffrey, 199-201
Kemnitz, Joe, 111
Kenyon, Cynthia, 94
Kirkwood, Thomas B.L., 35,
45
knockout technique, 76
Kolarz, Christian M., 230-32

L
Lakowski, Bernard, 93-94
Lander, Eric, 89-90
Lane, Mark, 149-50
language learning, 171
Lee, Anthony K., 68
life expectancies by coun-
try, 229
lions, 56
Liu, Danxia, 128
Liune, Victoria, 219-20
Living to 100 (Perls), 22. *See
also* Perls, Thomas
Longevity Assurance Gene

(LAG-1), 75-76
lotus seeds, 58
Lou Gehrig's disease, 126-28
Louisiana State University, 75
Louis XIV and Twenty Million Frenchmen (Goubert), 27
low density lipoproteins (LDLs), 99-100

M

McClearn, Gerald E., 194-96
McClintock, Barbara, 161
McCormick, Anna, 98
McCully, Kilmer S., 132-33
McDaniel, Geneva, 24-25
McEwen, Bruce, 219
McGill University (Montreal), 93-94
McKay, Clive, 103-4
Maddox, George, 20
malaria, 36
Manton, Kenneth G., 30, 228, 229
marsupial mice, 67-70
Martin, George, 97-98
Mayo Clinic, 142
Mayr, Ernest, 168, 179, 181
medical costs, 228-29
    older and cheaper, 29-31
Medicare, 10, 30, 31, 228
Mehta, Mehli, 168, 179-80, 181, 185-86
melatonin, 151-53

menopause, 17, 39-42, 214-15
mental abilities. *See* brains
Merriam, George, 148-49
Mestler, Gordon, 155-56
metabolic rates, 47-49, 51
Methuselah, 19
Metter, John, 221
mice, 47, 49-50
    caloric restriction experiments, 104-9
    marsupial mice, 67-70
    melatonin experiments, 152
    muscle-enhancing gene therapy, 139-40
mitochondria, 123-25
monkeys, 109-14. *See also* apes; chimpanzees
Morales, Arlene, 150
Mroczek, Daniel K., 230-32
muscle loss, 16
musclular dystrophies, 140

N

National Institute on Aging, 11, 23, 29, 113-14, 130-31, 144, 149, 196, 220-21
National Institutes of Health, 11
negative pleiotropy, 36
Nelson, Miriam, 16, 135-39, 144
nematodes, 14, 86-95
nephropathy, 117
Neurology, 199

neuropathy, 117
New England Centenarian
    Study, 23-24. *See also*
    Perls, Thomas
New England Journal of
    Medicine, 228
New Guinea, 42-44
New York Times, 12, 14
Nurses Health Study, 131-32

O

Odum, Eugene, 52
O'Keefe, Georgia, 167
one-hundred-year-olds, 19-
    20, 22-26, 28, 29, 32-33,
    35, 45-46, 232
opossums, 15, 59-65
Orentriech, Norman, 154-55
Osness, Wayne, 143-44
oxidation, 16, 100, 107-8,
    122-26, 129-31
oxygen consumption, 119-
    23

P

Pacific salmon, 66-67, 68,
    69-70
paradox of life, 123
Pearl, Raymond, 49
Perls, Thomas, 13-14, 22-25,
    27-29, 31-32, 34-35, 45-46
photosynthesis, 122
phyto chemicals, 129
Pierpaoli, Walter, 152
Pike, Malcom C., 33
Poon, Leonard, 25, 232

population of elderly, 227-
    28
Proceedings of the National
    Academy of Sciences,
    140
progeria, 96
prostate, 155
protein repair enzymes, 58
protozoa, 162, 163
p21 gene, 76

R

Raffray, André-François, 25-
    26
rate of living theory, 47-49,
    51
rats, 47, 103-4, 175-78
Regelson, Walter, 152
religious beliefs, 232
reproduction and child-
    bearing, 32, 35, 44-46
    first-time births and lon-
        gevity (humans), 44-46
    fission reproduction, 73-75
    fruit fly reproduction and
        aging, 78-83
    menopause, 39-42. *See*
        also menopause
    single-celled organisms,
        73-75
    stress of reproduction, 66-
        70
retinopathy, 117
retirement, 173-75
Rice, Bernice, 138
Rimm, Eric B., 131-32, 133

rockfish, 57

Rose, Michael, 14-15, 79-83, 86, 92

Roth, George, 113-14

Rubin, John, 18

Rubner, Max, 47-49

Rudman, Daniel, 147-48

Ruvkun, Gary, 95

S

Salthouse, Timothy A., 17, 182-88

Santa Fe Institute, 50

Sapelo Island opossums, 61-65

Sapolsky, Robert, 36, 69-70, 173-74, 198, 209-13, 224-25

Savannah River Ecology Laboratory (SC), 51-52

scaling theory, 49-51

Schaie, Warner, 17, 188-93, 194

Scheibel, Arnold, 169-75, 178

Schellenberg, George, 97-98

Schwartz, Robert, 148

Sedivy, John, 76-77

selective breeding, 79-83

self-repair, 37-38, 58, 64, 65-66

semelparity, 67-70

Shakespeare, William, 22, 216

Shapiro, Oscar, 168, 180, 181-82

Shay, Jerry, 164

Sheehy, Gail, 154-55

Shen-Miller, Jane, 58

Sherwin, Barbara, 17, 213-15

sickle cell anemia, 36

single-celled organisms, 73-75

  bacteria in amber, 71-73

  yeast, 72, 75, 77-78, 87, 88, 162

Smith, John Maynard, 78-79

smoking, 28, 31

Snowden, David, 202-5

Social Security, 10

Sohal, Raj, 15-16, 119-26, 128-29

spatial ability tests, 184-85, 189, 191

Staehelin, Hannes, 131

Stanford University, 87-88

Stock, Gregory, 13

Strandal, Angeline, 23-24

stress, 69, 92-93

  brain, effects on, 210-13, 224

  chronic stress, 78

  reproductive stress, 66-70

  Sapelo Island opossums, 61-65

stroke, 155

Sulston, John E., 88-89

Suzman, Richard M., 23, 228

Swedish Twin Registry, 194-96

Sweeney, H. Lee, 140
synapses, 170-71

T
telomeres and telomerase,
     161-66
Tennis, Letty, 218
Tenover, Joyce, 154
testosterone, 153-56
tigers, 56
Timagedine, 118
Tithonus, 108
Tolley, H. Dennis, 10, 30, 31
travel, 173
turtles, 52-56
Tyler, Robert, 86

U
Ulrich, Peter, 118

V
Vanity Fair, 154
Vaupel, James W., 229
vegetables, 128-29, 133
Verdi, Giuseppe, 167
vitalism, 48

vitamin B6, 131-33
vitamin C, 129-31
vitamin E, 129-31

W
Walford, Roy, 15, 103-9
Warner, Huber, 94-95
Waterston, Robert H., 88-89
Weinberg, Robert, 164-65
Weindruch, Richard, 109,
     110-13, 124
Werner, Otto, 96
Werner's Syndrome, 96-98
West, Geoffrey, 50-51
Westendorp, Rudi G.J., 45
whales, 39-40
Willis, Sherry, 188-91
Wilmoth, John, 33-34
wine, 128-29
Wisconsin Regional Primate
     Center, 110-14

Y
yeast, 72, 75, 77-78, 87, 88,
     162
Yen, Samuel S.C., 150

About the Author

FRED **WARSHOFSKY** is the author of ten books about science, medicine, and technology, most recently publishing *The Patent Wars, The Chip Wars,* and *The Control of Life.* He has also produced, written, and directed numerous television documentaries, including "Incredible Voyage," the first of television's excursions through the human body, "The Transplanted Heart," "The 21st Century," and "Science and Religion: Who Will Play God," and has won two Emmies, among other awards. For many years his commentaries on science and technology were a regular feature of PBS's "Nightly Business Report." He lives with his wife in North Carolina.